STP 1396

Synthetic Bioabsorbable Polymers for Implants

C. Mauli Agrawal, Jack E. Parr, and Steve T. Lin, editors

ASTM Stock Number: STP1396

ASTM
100 Barr Harbor Drive
PO Box C700
West Conshohocken, PA 19428-2959

Printed in the U. S. A.

Library of Congress Cataloging-in-Publication Data

Synthetic bioabsorbable polymers for implants
C. Mauli Agrawal, Jack E. Parr, and Steve T. Lin, editors.
p. cm.—(STP; 1396)
ASTM Stock Number: STP1396.
Includes bibliographical references.
ISBN 0-8031-2870-3
1. Polymers in medicine—Congresses. 2. Biomedical engineering—Congresses. 3. Biomedial materials—Congresses. I. Agrawal, C. Mauli (Chandra Mauli) II. Parr, Jack E. III. Lin, Steve T., 1947- IV. ASTM special technical publication; 1396.

R857.P6 S954 2000
610′.28—dc21

00-040612

Peer Review Policy

Each paper published in this volume was evaluated by two peer reviewers and at least one editor. The authors addressed all of the reviewers' comments to the satisfaction of both the technical editor(s) and the ASTM Committee on Publications.

To make technical information available as quickly as possible, the peer-reviewed papers in this publication were prepared "camera-ready" as submitted by the authors.

The quality of the papers in this publication reflects not only the obvious efforts of the authors and the technical editor(s), but also the work of the peer reviewers. In keeping with long-standing publication practices, ASTM maintains the anonymity of the peer reviewers. The ASTM Committee on Publications acknowledges with appreciation their dedication and contribution to time and effort on behalf of ASTM.

Printed in Scranton, PA
July 2000

Foreword

This publication, *Synthetic Bioabsorbable Polymers for Implants,* contains papers presented at the symposium of the same name held in Kansas City, Missouri, on 16–17 November 1999. The symposium was sponsored by ASTM Committee F4 on Medical and Surgical Materials and Devices. The symposium co-chairmen were C. Mauli Agrawal, The University of Texas Health Science Center, Jack E. Parr, Wright Medical Technology, Inc., and Steve T. Lin, Exactech, Inc.

Contents

Overview

Over the past decade, the use of synthetic bioabsorbable polymers in the field of medicine has grown steadily, and it is not uncommon today to find bioabsorbable devices commercially available for use as implants. The popularity of bioabsorbable polymers in medicine stems from the fact that implants fabricated from these materials are absorbed by the body over time. Moreover, the rate of absorption can be designed to meet the needs of the application. This is a significant advantage because nonabsorbable implants often have to be removed surgically after tissue healing has occurred. Also, most synthetic bioabsorbable polymers can easily be injection molded or extruded into a variety of shapes, which facilitates manufacturing and reduces cost.

As the awareness and the concomitant use of bioabsorbable devices increases, there is a need to address issues of novel and new applications, test and characterization techniques for raw materials and devices, efficacy, and long-term effects. The purpose of this symposium was to explore these issues, teach the latest developments in applications and test techniques, and promote the standardization of minimum requirements and test methodologies.

The papers included in this volume covered a variety of topics such as basic polymer properties and characterization, testing techniques, and tissue engineering. At the present time one of the most popular strategies used in tissue engineering is the implantation of a porous biodegradable scaffold at the defect site in the tissue. This scaffold may carry cells or other biomolecular signals to enable tissue regeneration. Synthetic biodegradable polymers are often used for the scaffolds, and thus, play an important role in tissue engineering. Also discussed were various aspects of biodegradable scaffolds. Lastly, bioabsorbable polymers are receiving attention as replacements for metallic fracture fixation devices and systems.

This STP provides an overview of the use of synthetic bioabsorbable polymers in the medical field at the present time. We predict that in the future such materials will play a very significant role as implants.

We would like to thank the ASTM staff (Dorothy Fitzpatrick, Teresa Cendrowska, and Annette Adams) for working so diligently on this project.

C. Mauli Agrawal
The University of Texas Health Science Center
San Antonio, Texas
Symposium Chairman and Editor

Jack Parr
Wright Medical Technology, Inc.
Arlington, Tennessee
Symposium Chairman and Editor

Steve Lin
Exactech
Gainesville, Florida
Symposium Chairman and Editor

John A. Disegi,[1] James W. Dwyer,[1] and Robert E. Fairer[1]

Mechanical Evaluation Of 70:30 Poly (L/DL-Lactide) Bone Screws After *In Vitro* Degradation

---

Reference: Disegi, J. A., Dwyer, J. W., and Fairer, R. E., **"Mechanical Evaluation of 70:30 Poly (L/DL-Lactide) Bone Screws After *In Vitro* Degradation,"** *Synthetic Bioabsorbable Polymers for Implants, ASTM STP 1396*, C. M. Agrawal, J. E. Parr, and S. T. Lin, Eds., American Society for Testing and Materials, West Conshohocken, PA, 2000.

Abstract: Controlled *in vitro* degradation testing is typically used to complement animal trials in order to understand the material, design, and fabrication factors that affect *in vivo* resorption rates of bioabsorbable implants. Resorbable 1.5 mm craniofacial bone screws were injection molded from amorphous 70:30 poly (L/DL-lactide) granules. The screws were vacuum dried, bulk packed, and gamma sterilized. Some of the screws were fully immersed in 7.4 pH phosphate buffer solution. The solutions were maintained at 37°C during short term exposure periods that extended to 8 weeks. Non-exposed control samples were stored in sterilized packages until the testing commenced. Stability testing was performed with rigid polyurethane foam to evaluate whether this test material was satisfactory for use in phosphate buffer solution.
Screw pull-out strength was measured in accordance with ASTM F 1691. Shear strength before and after *in vitro* degradation was analyzed by determining the maximum applied force required to shear the screw shaft when mounted in a specialized test fixture.

Keywords: degradation-surgical devices/applications, poly(L-lactic acid), testing methods-surgical implants, pull-out fixation strength, shear testing-medical materials/applications

---

Maxillofacial plates and screws produced from resorbable polymers have been evaluated by a number of researchers. The use of resorbable materials represents an ideal fracture fixation application since these implants are small in mass and subjected to relatively low stress during implantation. Initial fracture stabilization is extremely important because critical fracture healing of highly vascularized craniofacial regions may occur within a four to six week implantation period. Controlled *in vitro* degradation testing is commonly used to complement animal trials in order to understand the material, design, and fabrication factors that affect *in vivo* resorption rates. The present study

[1]Materials development manager, product development engineer, and mechanical test engineer, respectively, Synthes (USA) Technical Center, 1301 Goshen Parkway, West Chester, PA 19380.

evaluated the effect of *in vitro* phosphate buffer solution exposure on the mechanical property degradation of resorbable polylactide craniofacial bone screws. Pull-out and shear strength properties of resorbable bone screws were characterized since these attributes are important functional requirements that influence bone fracture stabilization and clinical performance.

Materials and Methods

High molecular weight $(C_3H_4O_2)_n$ polylactide compositions may be synthesized *[1]* by catalyzed ring opening polymerization of cyclic L, D, and DL lactide mixtures. DL lactide is a racemic mixture of the L(-) and D(+) isomeric forms. Nuclear magnetic resonance methods are used to analyze copolymers containing chemically different polymer units but stereoisomeric polylactide compositions are usually identified on the basis of their specific optical rotation *[2]*. Lactide polymers and copolymers may exhibit an amorphous solid state structure depending on the stereoisomeric ratios. The polylactide material utilized in the present study was amorphous 70:30 poly (L/DL-lactide) granular material with a maximum inherent viscosity of 6.5 dl/gm. Residual component limits for the 70:30 poly (L/DL-lactide) granules are shown in Table 1.

Table 1 – *Residual limits for 70:30 poly (L/DL-lactide) granules.*

Residual Component	Maximum Value
Monomer	0.5%
Solvents	0.1%
Water	0.5%
Sulfated Ash	0.1%
Heavy Metals	10 ppm
Tin	100 ppm

Amorphous 70:30 poly (L/DL-lactide) granules were obtained in nitrogen purged moisture resistant foil packages and stored at 6°C. Granules were vacuum dried for 16 hours at 70°C, resealed in nitrogen purged moisture resistant foil packages, and stored at 6°C. The packages were allowed to equilibrate to room temperature and granules were transferred under nitrogen to a hopper attached to injection molding equipment. The mold was heated and the granules were injection molded into 1.5 mm diameter maxillofacial bone screws. Injection molded screws were cooled, visually inspected for molding imperfections, and stored in a dessicator. Screws were visually and dimensionally inspected at finish to ensure the test specimens were uniform and consistent. Screw dimensions conformed to engineering drawings that were previously established for 1.5 mm diameter resorbable bone screws. The screws were vacuum dried, bulk packed, and gamma sterilized at a nominal dose of 25 kGy. Resorbable polylactide craniofacial bone screws and a resorbable bone plate are shown in Figure 1.

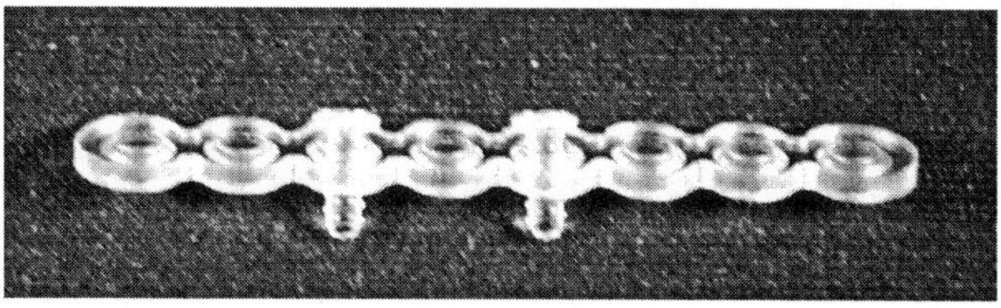

Figure 1 – *70:30 poly (L/DL-lactide) bone screws and plate (2.5X).*

Stability Testing

The use of cadaver bone as a test material to evaluate pull-out and shear properties of bone screws is problematic because of bone density and hardness nonuniformity. Polyurethane was evaluated as a possible test material for degradation testing since polyurethane foam is a recognized bone substitute material in ASTM Specification for Rigid Polyurethane Foam for Use as a Standard Material for Testing Orthopaedic Devices and Instruments (F 1839). Preliminary stability trials were performed with polyurethane foam to determine if degradation occcured in phosphate buffer solution and whether the test block material affected the pull-out of metallic bone screws. ASTM F 1839 Grade 40 polyurethane was selected since this material represents the highest density, pull-out strength, and shear modulus of the five grades that are covered in the ASTM standard. Titanium emergency screws with a 2.4 mm thread diameter were selected for the stability trials. It was felt that a pull-out force of sufficiently large magnitude might be needed in order to observe any small changes that may occur as a result of test block deterioration in the test solution. The blocks were drilled and tapped. Emergency 2.4 mm X 8 mm long titanium screws were fully inserted into the 16 mm wide X 16 mm long X 5 mm thick blocks. The screw insertion procedure conformed to ASTM Test Method for Driving Torque of Medical Bone Screws (F 117) and the torque test equipment has been described elsewhere *[3]*. Blocks with inserted titanium screws were fully immersed in 7.4 pH $\pm$ 0.2 phosphate buffer solution, also known as Sörensen buffer. The phosphate buffer solution was prepared according to the procedure outlined in Poly(L-lactide) Resins and Fabricted Forms for Surgical Implants – *In vitro* Degradation Testing (ISO 13781). Sörensen buffer consists of 1/15 mol/L potassium dihydrogen phosphate (KH_2PO_4 Solution A) plus 1/15 mol/L disodium hydrogen phosphate (Na_2HPO_4 Solution B) in sterile double-distilled water. The phosphate buffer solution was prepared from 18.2% volume fraction of Solution A and 81.8% volume fraction of Solution B. Solutions were maintained at 37°C during exposure periods of 4 weeks and 8 weeks. Control samples (0 hour immersion) were stored in packages until testing commenced. Eight control samples and eight samples from each exposure period were tested. Pull-out force was measured for the unexposed control samples and for the specimens immersed in Sörensen buffer. Mean, standard deviation, and Two-Tailed Student's T-Test ($p \leq 0.05$) statistical significance values were calculated.

Pull-Out Strength

Grade 40 blocks measuring 16 mm x 16 mm X 5 mm were drilled and tapped. Resorbable 1.5 mm X 6 mm long bone screws were inserted to a depth of 3.1 mm at 3

RPM according to procedures specified in ASTM F 117. Ten specimens were tested for each of the four *in vitro* conditioning treatments (0 hour control, 1 hour, 4 weeks, and 8 weeks). Resorbable bone screws were not allowed to dry out and they were tested immediately after each exposure period in Sörensen buffer. Control samples were stored in sterilized packages until testing commenced.

Pull-out strength testing was performed using a Model 810 MTS mechanical test system according to ASTM Test Method for Determining Axial Pull-Out Strength of Medical Bone Screws (F 1691). A Model 458 MTS electronic controller was used as a control and signal conditioning unit. Testing was conducted with the test system in displacement control at a displacement control rate of 5.0 mm per minute. Load versus displacement data was recorded with an X-Y recorder continuously monitoring the outputs from both the load cell and the hydraulic actuator mounted LVDT.

The test block was rigidly constrained in a collet attached to the test machine actuator. The screw head was captured in an articulated loading fixture that was attached to the test machine load cell. A view of the pull-out test fixture is shown in Figure 2.

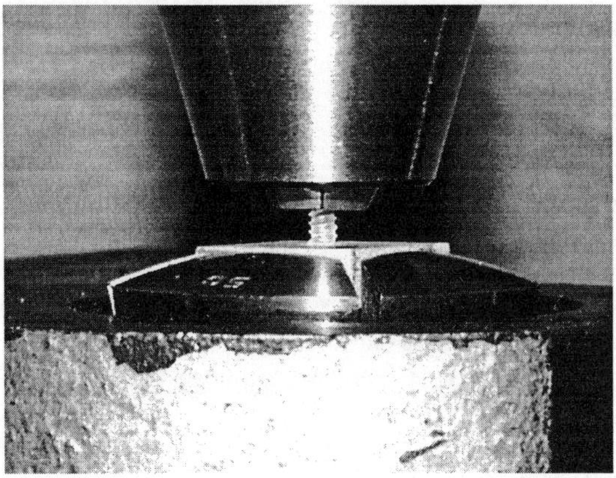

Figure 2 – *Pull-out test equipment with fixtured resorbable screw (1.7X).*

Shear Strength

Shear strength testing was performed with the 1.5 mm resorbable bone screws in accordance with a test protocol established by the project team. The test method used for this investigation measured the maximum applied shearing force needed to shear the screw shaft. The test equipment consisted of a Model 810 MTS mechanical test system and Model 458 MTS electronic controller. Shear tests were performed in displacement control at at a rate of 5.0 mm per minute. Load versus displacement data was recorded with an X-Y recorder continuously monitoring the outputs from both the load cell and the hydraulic actuator mounted LVDT.

The screw was placed in the shear fixture and the screw anchoring fixture was mounted on the test machine hydraulic actuator. A shearing blade was attached to the test equipment load cell. Ten 1.5 mm resorbable bone screws representing the 0 hour control period were shear tested in addition to ten specimens from each of the three *in vitro* immersion periods of 1 hour, 4 weeks, and 8 weeks. Resorbable bone screws were tested immediately after each exposure period in Sörensen buffer and were not allowed to dry out. Control samples were stored in sterilized packages until testing commenced.

Results and Discussion

Mean pull-out strength and standard deviation values for titanium and resorbable bone screws are compiled in Table 2.

Table 2 – *Pull-out results for titanium and resorbable screws inserted into Grade 40 polyurethane blocks.*

Immersion Period	Pull-out Strength (N) 2.4 mm Ti (n = 8)	1.5 mm Resorbable (n = 10)
Control	447 ± 47	37.3 ± 2.2
1 hour	---	27.7 ± 8.8
4 weeks	358 ± 33	37.4 ± 1.5
8 weeks	341 ± 22	33.8 ± 7.9

Mean pull-out values for the titanium screws were an order of magnitude larger than the resorbable screws. This result was expected based on the known differences in material properties and the larger size of the unalloyed titanium screws when compared to the amorphous polylactide screws. The Two-Tailed Student's T-Test ($p \leq 0.05$) indicated the 4 week and the 8 week pull-out strengths were significantly different when compared to the controls. The 4 week versus 8 week pull-out results were not significantly different. In general, titanium screws experienced a reduction in mean pull-out force over the 8 week timeframe. Stability test results indicated that the polyurethane foam experienced some form of degradation in Sörensen buffer as a function of exposure time. This material attribute was not unusual since biologically induced environmental stress cracking *[4]* has been reported for polyurethane materials. The specific mechanism responsible for the reduction in pull-out force was not identified but it was hypothesized that the combined action of the Sörensen buffer and superficial stress associated with screw insertion into the test blocks could account for the polyurethane degradation. Polyurethane test results indicated that a 24% reduction in mean pull-out strength was measured for titanium screws after 8 weeks immersion in phosphate buffer solution when compared to the mean control value.

The mean pull-out strengths of the resorbable bone screws were essentially unchanged after exposure testing. The one hour data was not statistically compared to the control because of the brief immersion time. The control vs. 4 week, control vs. 8 week, and 4 week vs. 8 week resorbable pull-out results were not significantly different but the data showed some scatter as a function of time. The reason for the scatter is unknown but may be related to the test setup, random error, and/or localized variations in the reaction rate of polyurethane when exposed to the buffer solution. Regardless of the factors responsible for the data scatter, an important observation was documented for the pull-out failure mode of the bioresorbable screws. The screws did not fail by pull-out from the polyurethane test block material. The screw heads of the resorbable screws fractured due to tensile failure. This observation indicated that the resorbable screw pull-out strength was not significantly influenced by the polyurethane foam deterioration that occurred during the test periods. Stability test results suggested that polyurethane foam is a suitable test material for examining the mechanical properties of 70:30 poly (L/DL-lactide) bone screws following exposure to phosphate buffer solution for 8 weeks. The amorphous lactide stereopolymer examined in this study has a very slow *in vitro* and *in vivo* resorption rate and the testing protocol may not be suitable for other polymer compositions with different resorption rates.

Mean shear load, standard deviation, and % mean shear load retention for the 1.5 resorbable screws are shown in Table 3.

Table 3 - *Shear strength results for 1.5 mm resorbable screws.*

Immersion Period	Mean Shear Load (N) (n = 10)	Shear Load Retention[1] (%)
Control	83.1 ± 5.6	---
1 hour	78.7 ± 8.4	95 ± 10
4 weeks	69.6 ± 5.5	84 ± 7
8 weeks	72.5 ± 6.3	87 ± 8

[1] Shear load retention (%) = Shear load (N) X 100 / Mean control shear load (N)

Shear strength data for the one hour immersion period was not statistically analyzed due to the short exposure time. Student's T-Test analysis indicated the control vs. 4 week and control vs. 8 week resorbable shear strength results were significantly different while the 4 week vs. 8 week results were not significantly different. Data scatter was also observed for mean shear strength results.

Claes et. al. *[5]* investigated the mechanical properties of 70:30 poly (L/DL-lactide) implants after *in vitro* phosphate-buffered saline (PBS) exposure testing at 37°C. In the referenced report, 4.0 mm diameter non-threaded pins were ethylene oxide sterilized and 3-point bend tested after short term and long term PBS exposure periods. Their results indicated that no decrease in bending rigidity was experienced after 8 weeks exposure. Scatter in the bend test data was observed at 1, 2, 4, and 8 week exposure intervals. This observation suggested that test scatter associated with brief immersion times may be related to random measurement errors during the timeframe when *in vitro* resorption has not significantly influenced mechanical property degradation. Implant geometry, sterilization method, physiological soaking solution, and mechanical test methods were different in the Claes paper. However, scatter in the mechanical property values after short term exposure intervals and retention of mechanical properties at 8 weeks exposure were in agreement with the trends observed for the pull-out test results obtained in the present study.

Conclusions

1. Rigid polyurethane foam demonstrated some degradation during eight weeks exposure in phosphate buffer solution but the test blocks appeared to be satisfactory for *in-vitro* degradation testing of resorbable 70:30 poly (L/DL-lactide) craniofacial bone screws.

2. The pull-out strengths of 1.5 mm resorbable screws were not significantly different than unexposed control samples after 4 week and 8 week immersion periods while screw shear strengths were reduced during this time interval.

3. Data scatter was observed in the present study but other researchers have also reported scatter in the mechanical properties of 70:30 poly(L/DL-lactide) implants after relatively brief *in vitro* exposure to physiological test solution.

References

[1] Entenmann, G., "Resorbable Polyesters: Composition, Properties, Applications," *Biodegradable Implants in Orthopaedic Surgery-2nd International Workshop on Implant Materials*, G. O. Hofmann, Ed., Technik+ Kommunikation Verlags GmbH, Berlin, 1990, pp. 14-19.

[2] Bendix, D. R., Internal Report on "Analytical Methods Used for the Characterization of Resorbable Polymers," Boehringer Ingelheim KG, Ingelheim, Germany, 1997, p. 1.

[3] Disegi, J. A., Fairer, R. E., "Torsional Properties of Ti-15Mo Bone Screws," *Transactions 21st Annual Meeting Society for Biomaterials*, San Francisco, CA, 1995, p. 351.

[4] CT Biomaterials Fact Sheet for ChronoFlex® AL, Woburn, MA, Number A:\CFAL.796.

[5] Claes, L., Rehm K., and Hutmacher, D., Internal Report on "Project Polypin" (German Translation), Biovision, Freiburg-Umkirch, Germany, 1993, pp. 7-17.

Jacqueline M. Allan,[1] Jacob A. Flagle,[1] Jonathan D. Kline,[1] R. Larry Dooley,[2] and Shalaby W. Shalaby[1]

Evaluation of Adhesive and Absorption Properties for Absorbable Tissue Adhesives

---

Reference: Allan, J. M., Flagle, J. A., Kline, J. D., Dooley, R. L., and Shalaby, S. W., "**Evaluation of Adhesive and Absorption Properties for Absorbable Tissue Adhesives**," *Synthetic Bioabsorbable Polymers for Implants, ASTM STP 1396*, C. M. Agrawal, J. E. Parr, and S. T. Lin, Eds., American Society for Testing and Materials, West Conshohocken, PA, 2000.

Abstract: Absorbable tissue adhesives for wound repair have gained interest in recent years compared with traditional devices for wound closure such as sutures and staples. While the demand for tissue adhesives continues to increase, *in vitro* methods for their evaluation remain scarce. The lack of a widely accepted method for evaluation of tissue adhesives and the availability of a family of novel absorbable tissue adhesive systems provided an incentive to develop a test method for assessing the two key parameters of candidate adhesives, namely adhesive strength and absorption. This report describes a new method for determining the absorption characteristics and adhesive strength of methoxypropyl cyanoacrylate-oxalate formulations.

Keywords: tissue adhesive, adhesion, absorption, methoxypropyl cyanoacrylate, MPC

Introduction

In an earlier communication Poly-Med, Inc. reported preliminary data on the use of new methods for evaluating the adhesive properties of absorbable tissue adhesives based on methoxypropyl cyanoacrylate (MPC) [*1*, *2*]. The compositions of these adhesives were described earlier by Linden and Shalaby [*3*]. Methods used to evaluate these materials included an *in vitro* goat skin model, nylon film peel test, and cotton fabric peel test [2]. Based on data obtained by these methods, the cotton fabric peel test was identified as the most promising and reliable method for evaluation of the adhesive properties of MPC systems. In the current study, the cotton fabric peel test was applied to the evaluation of MPC based adhesives containing oxalate modifiers (MPC-OX) with different absorption profiles. In addition, a new method was developed to determine the absorption characteristics of these adhesives.

---

[1]Manager of bioengineering and materials research, research engineer, staff scientist, director of research and development, respectively, Poly-Med, Inc., Westinghouse Rd., Pendleton, SC, 29670.

[2]Dept. Chair, Bioengineering Department, Clemson University, Clemson, SC, 29634.

Materials and Methods

Adhesive Properties

Plain weave cotton fabric (306 grams/m^2) was cut into swatches measuring 2.5 cm by 8.0 cm. The fabric was conditioned by submerging in phosphate buffer (pH = 7.2) and air drying for 25 min. MPC based adhesive formulations containing varying amounts of an oxalate modifier were applied over a 2.5 cm by 6 cm area on one swatch, and a mating sample was aligned on top; 350 µL of the adhesive formulation was used for each test sample. The assembled samples were cured beneath a 1 200 g weight for one minute and then were further cured on the bench top for 2 min. or 60 min. A schematic of the assembled test samples is shown in Figure 1.

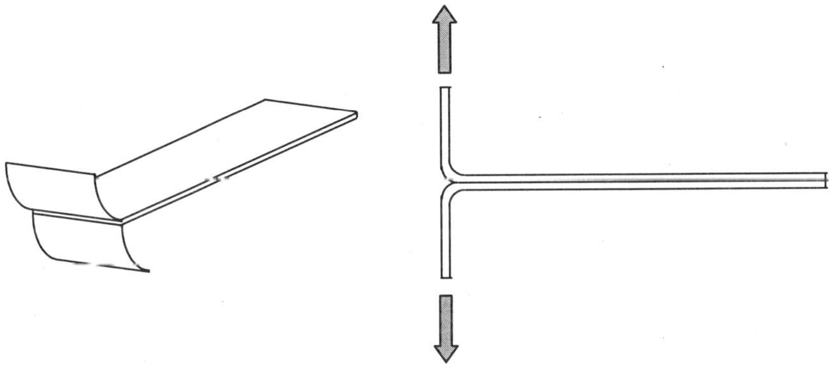

Figure 1—*Schematic representation of assembled test specimen.*

The adhesive properties of the absorbable MPC-OX formulations were determined by testing the assembled samples in tension on an MTS 858 Minibionix universal testing apparatus. The unadhered flaps of each specimen were secured into tensile grips, and the force required to separate the fabric at a displacement rate of 5.0 cm/min was measured. The average load after the initial peak was used to calculate the average peel strength of the adhesive which was reported as the force required to separate the samples divided by the width of the sample (in this case 2.5 cm). Five adhesive formulations were tested at 2 min. and 60 min. cure times. For each formulation and cure time, four samples per group were tested.

Absorption Characteristics

The absorption characteristics of a representative MPC-OX formulation were determined for samples stored in phosphate buffer. Thin disc shaped samples were prepared by applying 300 μL of a 5% sodium bicarbonate solution to a polymethyl methacrylate plate. Ten microliters of the MPC-OX adhesive formulation were then pipetted onto the sodium bicarbonate pool. Upon contact with the liquid, the adhesive formulation cured and formed a thin disc measuring approximately 10 mm in diameter. Control MPC discs were similarly prepared. Cured discs were rinsed in distilled water, dried under reduced pressure at 37°C, and weighed prior to initiation of the absorption study. Five samples for each formulation were incubated in phosphate buffer (pH = 7.4) at 37°C for a period of 75 days. At the conclusion of the study, remaining portions of the samples were removed from the buffer and were dried under reduced pressure at 37°C. The final weight of the sample was recorded, and the mass loss was reported as a percentage of the initial sample weight.

Results and Discussion

Adhesive Properties

The cotton fabric peel test was used for evaluation of the adhesive properties of several MPC-OX adhesives. The results of these tests are presented in Table 1 as averages with corresponding standard deviations. Overall, the test method allows for discrimination of the adhesive properties of the various formulations. For the formulations tested, adhesive strength increased with curing time with the exception of Formulation 1 in which the difference in strength between the two curing times was not significant. In the future, a minimally acceptable adhesive strength should be defined for the 2 min. time period to ensure secure wound closure upon application of the tissue adhesive.

Table 1—*Adhesive strength as measured by the cotton fabric peel test.*

	Adhesive Strength, N/m	
Formulation	2 min. Cure	60 min. Cure
1	227 ± 73	193 ± 21
2	326 ± 80	842 ± 131
3	741 ± 277	801 ± 147
4	825 ± 244	1,239 ± 64
5	480 ± 54	636 ± 135

Absorption Profile

Results of the absorption study are presented as the percent mass loss in Table 2; values are presented as averages and corresponding standard deviations. As expected, the adhesive formulation containing the absorbable modifier exhibited a significantly faster absorption rate than the unmodified control.

Table 2—*Absorption of MPC and MPC-OX formulations after incubation in phosphate buffer (pH 7.4, 37°C) for 75 days.*

Adhesive	Mass Loss, %
MPC	55 ± 3
MPC-OX	80 ± 4

Conclusion

The cotton fabric peel test is a reliable and reproducible method for evaluating the adhesive properties of absorbable tissue adhesives. Through the addition of varying amounts of an absorbable modifier, the adhesive properties of MPC can be tailored to specific applications. Addition of the absorbable modifier increases the absorption rate of the adhesive formulation by a significant degree as demonstrated by the results of the absorption study.

Acknowledgement

This work was supported by DOD grant no. DAMD-17-98-1-8654.

References

[1] Linden, Jr., C.L. and Shalaby, S.W., "Performance of Modified Cyanoacrylate Composition as Tissue Adhesives for Soft and Hard Tissues," *Journal of Biomedical Materials Research (Applied Biomaterials)*, Vol. 38, No. 4, 1997, p. 348.

[2] Flagle, J.A., Kline, J.D., Allan, J.M. and Shalaby, S.W., "Absorbable Tissue Adhesives in Skin Wound Repair," *Transactions of the Society for Biomaterials*, Vol. 22, 1999, p. 376.

[3] Linden, Jr., C.L. and Shalaby, S.W., "Absorbable Tissue Adhesives," U.S. Patent 5,350,798, 1994.

Yves Marois,[1] Ze Zhang,[1] Michel Vert,[2] Xiaoyan Deng,[1] Robert W. Lenz,[3] and Robert Guidoin[1]

Bacterial Polyesters for Biomedical Applications : In vitro and in vivo Assessments of Sterilization, Degradation Rate and Biocompatibility of Poly (β-hydroxyoctanoate) (PHO)

Reference: Marois, Y., Zhang, Z., Vert, M., Deng, X., Lenz, R. W., and Guidoin R., **"Bacterial Polyesters for Biomedical Applications: In vitro and In vivo Assessments of Sterilization, Degradation Rate and Biocompatibility of Poly (β-hydroxyoctanoate) (PHO)"** *Synthetic Bioabsorbable Polymers for Implants, ASTM STP 1396,* C. M. Agrawal, J. E. Parr, and S. T. Lin, Eds., American Society for Testing and Materials, West Conshohocken, PA, 2000.

Abstract : Poly (β-hydroxyalkanoates) (PHAs) are bacterial polyesters with chemical and physical properties that make them suitable for medical applications. They are obtained by fermentation techniques, are biodegradable and may be metabolized into normal constituents of the body. A PHA produced by *Pseudomonas oleovorans* has generated a random copolymer called poly (β-hydroxyoctanoate) (PHO) having elastomeric properties and displaying lower crystallinity and less rigidity than poly (β-hydroxybutyrate) (PHB). As part of an extensive study, we compared the effects of two methods of sterilization on the physical and structural characteristics of PHO, studied the mechanism and degradation rate of PHO *in vitro* over a 24-month period in physiological media and finally, investigated the biocompatibility and degradation rate of PHO *in vivo* as a new sealant for the polyester arterial prosthesis. Results have shown that the physical and structural properties of PHO were well-preserved after ethylene oxide sterilization, whereas gamma radiation caused random chain scission and physical cross-linking. *In vitro* incubation studies demonstrated that the degradation rate of PHO films in water or isoosmotic PBS is a very slow hydrolytic process exceeding two years. *In vivo*, PHO showed good biocompatibility in terms of tissue enzymatic activity and cellular reactions. Degradation was slow and exhibited similar rate as that observed *in vitro*. As a sealant in a polyester arterial prosthesis, PHO contributed to the impermeabilization of the graft wall and to the development of an internal collagenous capsule with a confluent endothelium secreting prostacyclin.

Keywords : polyhydroxy alkanoates, polyhydroxy octanoate, PHO, sterilization, degradation, biocompatibility, in vivo studies, arterial grafts, sealant

---

[1] Professors, Institut des biomatériaux du Québec, Hôpital St-François d'Assise, 10, rue de l'Espinay, Québec, Canada G1L 3L5

[2] Research Director, CRBA, UPRESA CNRS 5473, Université Montpellier 1, Faculté de Pharmacie, 15 avenue Charles Flahault, 34060, Montpellier, Cedex 2, France.

[3] Professor Emeritus, Polymer Science and Engineering, Silvio O. conte National Center for Polymer Research, University of Massachusetts, Amherst, MA, 01003-4530

Introduction

Poly (β-hydroxy alkanoates) (PHAs) are very promising bacterial polyesters with chemical and physical properties that make them suitable for biomedical applications *[1]*. This class of polymer is synthetized by bacteria in response to environmental stresses in an excess of carbon source, and its presence in the bacteria as intracellular granules serves as carbon and energy reserves. They are easily obtained by fed-batch fermentation processes and their composition determined by the type and concentrations of the carbon sources available during polymer synthesis.

Known members of this family of aliphatic polyesters are the poly (β-hydroxy butyrate) (PHB) and copolymer poly (β-hydroxy butyrate) / poly (β-hydroxy valerate) (PHB / HV) which have been successfully used for biomedical applications such as patches for arterial and pericardial repair *[2,3]* and guided bone regeneration *[4]*. However, these short chain-length PHAs are too brittle and rigid and may not be the best choice for vascular application. The poly (β-hydroxy octanoate) (PHO) produced by *Pseudomonas oleovorans* using sodium n-octanoic acid as the carbon source, is an elastomeric random copolymer (C_8 in majority) which may be best suited for arterial graft impregnation and which was therefore used in the present investigation as a substrate on a polyester arterial prosthesis.

As part of an extensive study, we 1) compared the effects of two methods of sterilization on the physical and structural characteristics of PHO, 2) studied the mechanism and degradation rate of PHO in vitro over a 24-month period in physiological media, 3) investigated the biocompatibility and degradation rate of PHO in vivo as a novel sealant for the polyester arterial prosthesis and 4) evaluated its healing behaviour after one month of implantation as an arterial substitute in the canine abdominal aorta.

Materials and Methods

Preparation of the PHO Films

Poly (β-hydroxy octanoate) (PHO) was biosynthesized in a fed-batch fermentation process using *Pseudomonas oleovorans* with sodium octanoate as the sole carbon source. When the polymer reached the early stationary growth phase, it was extracted from lyophilized cells using chloroform and precipitated in methanol *[5]*. Thereafter, the obtained material underwent several extraction and precipitation procedures. The repeating unit composition of the PHO obtained after preparation was 97% C_8 and 3% C_6, as determined by acid-catalyzed methanolysis using gas chromatography.

Films were first obtained by casting, using a chloroform solution of PHO at a concentration of 0.16 g/mL on a glass dish, then allowed to crystallize at room temperature for 2 to 3 weeks, at which time the solvent was believed to be completely removed from the films *[5]*. Samples of the PHO-cast films measuring 2.5 x 2.5 cm were cut with a scalpel, displaying a mean thickness of 0.12 ± 0.02 mm s.d. and a mean weight of 80.7 ± 13.2 mg s.d.

Sterilization Procedures

Ethylene Oxide Sterilization - Ethylene oxide sterilization was carried out using a cold cycle in a Castle 5 gas chamber (Getinge-Castle, Montréal, Qc, Canada). This cold cycle involved an ethylene oxide exposure time of 8 hours while maintaining the initial preheat, gas exposure, and final air purge conditions at 38°C with 65% humidity. Following sterilization, the films were air-dried for a minimum period of one week at room temperature.

Gamma Radiation - Gamma radiation sterilization was performed in a Gamma cell 220 cobalt 60 irradiation unit (Atomic Energy of Canada Ltd, Ottawa, Qc, Canada) at a dose of 2.5 Mrad in air and at room temperature.

Hydrolytic Incubation Study

The PHO-cast films were weighed, then placed in small cap-sealed glass bottles and immersed in either deionized filtered water (pH 7.0) or isoosmotic phosphate buffer saline (PBS) (0.13M; pH 7.4). To prevent bacterial contamination during the incubation, both aqueous media contained 0.05% sodium azide (NaN_3). The films were incubated without agitation in a thermostatically controlled oven set at 37°C for periods of 1, 3, 6, 12 and 24 months. Three PHO samples were analyzed for each incubation time and medium.

Physical Characterization

Water Absorption and Weight Loss Measurements - At each prescheduled incubation time, the films were removed from the bottles, gently placed on filter paper and immediately weighed to determine the amount of absorbed water in each film. They were then immersed several times in deionized water and dried in a vacuum oven at room temperature for 72 hours, at which time the weight remained constant. The films were weighed again to assess the mass loss as a function of incubation time and then tested in a dry state.

Mechanical Properties - Tensile strength measurements were carried out on an Instron Universal tensile tester, model 1130 (Instron Canada, Burlington, ON, Canada) fitted with a 100 g load cell and flat, rubber-faced jaws. A cross-head speed of 100 mm/min was used to extend the one cm-long dumbel-shaped specimens having an initial gauge length of 5 mm to failure *[6]*. The tensile strength was recorded and averaged for three tests for each sample after incubation.

Chemical Analyses

Fourier Transform Infrared Spectroscopy (FTIR) - Infrared studies were performed with a Nicolet Magna 550 Fourier transform infrared spectrometer (Nicolet, Madison, WI, USA) with a DTGS (deuterated triglycine sulphate) detector and a germanium-coated KBr beamsplitter. Two hundred scans were acquired with an optical retardation of 0.25 cm, and were triangularly apodized and Fourier transformed to yield a 4 cm^{-1} resolution. The attenuated total reflectance mode was used to obtain the infrared spectra of the PHO with a Split Pea attachment (Harrick Scientific

Corporation, Ossining, NY, USA) equipped with a hemispherical, 3 mm-diameter silicon internal reflection element (IRE). The IRE is bevelled along the edge of its flat surface to provide a sampling area slightly larger than the 150-200 μm diameter hot spot on the crystal.

Differential Scanning Calorimetry (DSC) - Thermograms depicting the glass transition (Tg) and melting (Tm) temperatures and the heat of fusion (ΔH) were obtained using a DSC-7 thermal analyzer (Perkin Elmer, Montréal, QC, Canada). PHO samples weighing approximately 10 mg each were heated from -100 to 120°C at a scanning rate of 10°C min^{-1}, using liquid nitrogen as the coolant and helium as the protective atmosphere. Indium and pure water were used to calibrate the instrument. Three measurements were made to obtain the average Tg, Tm and ΔH of the PHO incubated in either water or PBS at each incubation time.

Size Exclusion Chromatography (SEC) - Size exclusion chromatography was used to determine the molecular weight of each PHO sample. Each specimen was dissolved in a pre-filtered (0.45 and 0.22 μm) chromatograph grade tetrahydrofuran (THF) solvent at a concentration of 0.5% (w/v). Following filtration through a 0.45 μm nylon membrane filter (CSC, Montréal, QC, Canada), 300 μL of the PHO solution was injected through a syringe-loading sample injector (Rheodyne Model 7125) into a Waters Millipore® model 590 pump (Millipore Canada Ltd., Waters, Ville St-Laurent, QC, Canada) operating at a flow rate of 1.0 mL/min. The pump was fitted with an Ultrastyragel™ linear column (2000 - 4m, Millipore Canada Ltd., Waters, Ville St-Laurent, QC, Canada) and a Shodex® KF804 column (size exclusion limit of 4 x 10^5) (Showa Denko KK, Millipore Canada Ltd.). A Dawn® model F laser photometer and a Wyatt/Optilab 903 interferometric refractometer (Wyatt Technology Corporation, Santa Barbara, CA, USA) were connected to the column in series for the detection of molecular weight. The Dawn/RI delay value was measured using monodisperse polystyrene standards. The dn/dc value of the PHO solution was measured at 0.067 mL/g and was used as the input parameter to calculate the molecular weight.

In Vivo Biocompatibility and Degradation Study

Vascular Graft Selection and Preparation – Three (3) experimental vascular prostheses were selected for the present study. The reference polyester graft was the VP1200K ERS Dacron® arterial prosthesis (Vascutek Ltd., Inchinnan, Scotland). It is a warp-knit arterial prosthesis made of texturized polyester yarns knitted in a two-bar reverse lock-knit structure. The experimental grafts were impregnated with PHO using a 20% chloroform solution (w/v). The graft segments were first soaked and dried four times in the PHO solution, then allowed to stabilize at room temperature for three weeks, at which time, the chloroform is believed to be completely removed from the grafts. [5] They were then sterilized either by ethylene oxide gas, using a cold cycle at 38°C, with 65% humidity and an exposure time of 8 hours, followed by proper aeration for one week at room temperature, or by gamma radiation at a dose of 2.5 Mrad in air at room temperature.

In Vivo Implantation - One hundred and forty four (144) female Sprague-Dawley rats, each weighing between 200 and 250 g (Charles River Inc., St-Constant, Québec, Canada), were divided into four groups: one sham-operated control group (trauma without implant), and three experimental groups, one for each experimental vascular graft studied. Four (4) rats were used for each of the following prescheduled implantation periods : 2, 5, 7, 10, 15, 30, 60, 120 and 180 days. Following isoflurane gas anesthesia (Forane®, Anaquest, Pointe-Claire, Québec, Canada), one 2 cm-long graft segment was implanted subcutaneously in the back of each rat. Briefly, the back region was shaved and the skin disinfected with gluconate chlorexidrine (Proviodine®, Rougier, Chambly, Québec, Canada). A 2 cm-long incision was then performed and the graft specimen inserted. The incision was immediately closed and sutured with 3-0 monofilament polypropylene sutures (Prolene®, Ethicon, Peterborough, Ontario, Canada), and the area disinfected again. After awakening, the animal was sent to the animal facility, fed an unrestricted diet and treated according to the Canadian Council on Animal Care Regulations.

Graft Harvesting - At the sacrifice, the graft specimens and surrounding tissue were removed and divided into two separate samples for the determination of enzyme activity and for histology. For the ethylene oxide and gamma-sterilized PHO grafts, a third sample was retained for chemical analysis.

Quantification of Enzyme Activities - For the alkaline phosphatase determination, the graft specimens were weighed separately, soaked in a cold glycine buffer (50 mM, pH 10.5) and homogenized. Following centrifugation, the supernatant liquid was removed and immediately tested for alkaline phosphatase activity. Briefly, the substrate (p-nitrophenyl phosphate) (Sigma Chemical Co., St. Louis, MO, USA) was dissolved at a concentration of 0.4 mg/mL in the same buffer, and 1 mL of this solution was mixed with 200 μl of supernatant and allowed to react for 30 minutes at 37°C. The reaction was then stopped with 1 mL of 0.02 N NaOH and the optical density was read at 400 nm using a Spectronic 21 spectrophotometer (Milton Roy Inc., Rochester, NY, USA). Alkaline phosphatase of porcine origin (Sigma Chemical Co.) was used to determine the standard curve. For the acid phosphatase assay, the graft specimens were weighed separately, soaked in a cold citrate buffer (50 mM, pH 5.0) and homogenized. Following centrifugation, the supernatant liquid was removed and immediately tested for acid phosphatase activity using the same method described above. Acid phosphatase of wheat germ origin (Sigma) was used as the standard curve. In the present study, alkaline and acid phosphatase were selected because they are greatly secreted by polymorphonuclear cells (alkaline phosphatase) and macrophages (acid phosphatase) during the inflammatory response to biomaterials implanted in the body. [7]

Histology - The graft specimens were harvested and immediately fixed in a 10% formaline solution for several days prior to processing. They were then embedded in paraffin wax, cut into 5 μm-thick sections, stained with hematoxylin, phloxine, safran (HPS), and Masson's trichrome separately, and observed on an Axiophot light microscope (Zeiss, Oberkochen, Germany). The type and the intensity of the inflammatory reaction were determined and the extent of healing was analyzed in terms of collagen synthesis, coating presence and degree of tissue infiltration into the implant. The PHO graft specimens were also embedded in L.R. White resin to preserve the polymer during histological processing. The samples were dehydrated in a series of alcohol-graded solutions and immersed overnight in a LR White-alcohol solution at -20°C. They were then embedded in pure L.R. White resin for a few hours at -20°C prior to being cast at room temperature in gelatin-coated molds with caps to prevent O_2 contact. One and ½ μm-thick sections were cut on an ultramicrotome and stained with Azure 2 and toluidine blue.

Chemical Analyses - Specimens from the ethylene oxide and gamma-sterilized PHO-impregnated grafts were cleaned of excess tissue (using plastic tweezers) and cut into two separate samples for DSC and SEC studies to assess the rate of degradation of the PHO during implantation. For DSC, the PHO was analyzed while still inside the prosthetic skeleton. For SEC, the PHO was removed from the polyester graft by solubilization in chloroform for one hour followed by vigorous extraction in a solution of methanol (50%): chloroform (1:3) at room temperature. The bottom phase (chloroform containing PHO) was then collected, and allowed to dry *in vacuo* in glass vials for three weeks at room temperature prior to testing.

In Vivo Healing Behaviour of PHO-Impregnated Grafts

Animal Selection - Eight (8) adult mongrel dogs of either sex, each weighing between 20 and 25kg, were selected and treated according to the Canadian Council on Animal Care regulations. Prior to surgery, routine hematological tests were performed, including hematocrit, leukocyte and platelet counts, platelet aggregation and thromboelastography.

Surgery - The dogs were fasted for 24 hours prior to surgery. They were administered an I.M. premedication bolus of 0.05 mg/kg of atropine sulfate (MTC Pharmaceuticals, Cambridge, ON, Canada) and 0.1 mg/kg of acepromazine maleate (Atravet®, Ayerst Laboratories, Montréal, QC, Canada). They were then anesthesized with 10 mg/kg I.V. of sodium thiopental (Pentothal®, Abbott Laboratoires, Montréal, QC, Canada), intubated and mechanically ventilated. Isoflurane gas (Aerrane®, Janssen, North York, ON, Canada) was used to maintain anesthesia as required. Intravenous infusions of Ringer's lactate was injected to compensate for dehydration during surgery. The abdomen was shaved and the skin disinfected with Hibitane® chlorhexidrine gluconate (Ayerst) and 10% Proviodine® iodine USP topical solution (Rougier, Chambly, QC, Canada). A midline lower abdominal incision was performed and the abdominal aorta was isolated from the renal arteries to the aortic trifurcation. After collateral ligation, the animals were given 0.5 mg/kg of intravenous heparin (Hepalean®, Organon Teknika Inc., Toronto, ON, Canada) at least 5 minutes prior to vascular clamping. Five (5) cm long, six mm in diameter preclotted VP1200K ERS arterial prosthesis and the PHO-impregnated VP1200K ERS graft sterilized by ethylene oxide were anastomosed using 4/0 braided polyester sutures (Ticron®) Upon complete hemostasis, the abdomen was closed in layers using 2/0 Vicryl® and PDS monofilament sutures, and the skin was stapled. Upon awakening, the animals were returned to their cages and fed an unrestricted standard diet. They also received 0.2 mg/kg of butorphanol tartrate (Torbugesic®, Ayerst) for 3 days as a post-op analgesic.

Pathological Studies - After one month of implantation, the experimental grafts were harvested, rinsed in heparinized saline, opened longitudinally and photographed with a Dental camera (Yashica Canada, Mississauga, ON, Canada) and a Tessovar macrophotography optical system (Carl Zeiss, Oberkochen, Germany). Representative specimens from the proximal, medial and distal regions were selected for pathological analysis and were subdivided into two samples. The first halves underwent scanning electron microscopic studies by being post-fixed in a 2% isotonic buffered glutaraldehyde solution and in osmium tetroxide, then dried by immersion in a series of aqueous solutions of increasing ethanol concentration, followed by critical point drying, with liquid CO_2 as the transfer medium. The specimens were then coated with gold and examined in a Jeol JSM 35 CF scanning electron microscope (Soquelec Ltd., Montréal, QC, Canada) at a 15 kV accelerating voltage. The second halves samples for histologic study were embedded in paraffin, and 5 μm-thick sections were cut and stained with hematoxylin-eosin, Weigert, Masson's trichrome and Dahl's stain.

Prostacyclin and Thromboxane A_2 Secretion Assays - Fresh segments (1 cm^2) were removed from both proximal, distal, medial, and regions of each arterial grafts and immediately incubated in 50 mM Tris-HCL buffer for 30 min at 37°C. Aliquots of buffer were then quick frozen and subsequently tested for PGI_2 and TXA_2 secretion using 6-keto-PGF_1 and thromboxane B_2 radioimmunoassay kits, respectively (New England Nuclear, Boston MA, USA). Each sample was tested in duplicate and the results expressed as the mean PGI_2/TXA_2 ratio for each graft region of each type of grafts. The abdominal aortas served as controls.

Statistical Analysis

Results are expressed as the mean ± standard deviation. Groups were compared using the one way ANOVA test. Statistical significance was obtained with a p value of < 0.05.

Results

Effects of sterilization

Tensile Properties - The tensile strength of the PHO-cast films sterilized by EO (1.74 ± 0.06 kPa) was not significantly different from that of the PHO-cast films prior to sterilization, which was 1.55 ± 0.32 kPa. In contrast, a significant increase in tensile strength of 2.15 ± 0.15 kPa was recorded following gamma sterilization.

Differential Scanning Calorimetry - The results of the thermal analysis of the PHO-cast films before and after sterilization by ethylene oxide gas or gamma radiation demonstrate that the PHO films sterilized by EO gas showed no significant change in the glass transition or melting temperatures nor in the heat of fusion when compared to PHO-cast films prior to sterilization. However, while the Tm of the PHO films sterilized by gamma radiation decreased to 46.1°C, the Tm of the PHO films sterilized by EO gas remained at 47.3°C. Finally, the heat of fusion of the gamma-sterilized PHO increased to 19.6 J/g, compared to 16.1 J/g for the PHO-cast films before sterilization.

Molecular Weight Measurements - Figure 1 presents the results of the molecular weight of the PHO-cast films before sterilization and those sterilized by either ethylene oxide gas or gamma radiation. Sterilization of the PHO by EO induced a slight decrease in both the weight average ($\overline{M}w$) and the number average ($\overline{M}n$) molecular weights which did not exceed 5%. A significant reduction of 17% in $\overline{M}w$ and 25% in $\overline{M}n$ were recorded following gamma sterilization.

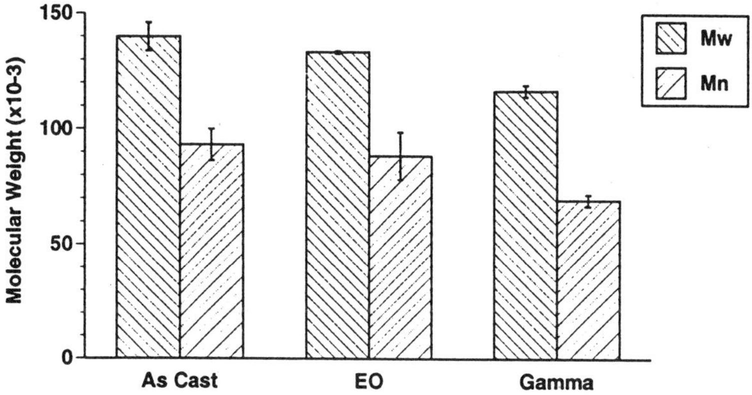

Figure 1 : Molecular weight results of PHO before and after ethylene oxide (EO) gas or gamma sterilization.

In Vitro Hydrolytic Study

Water Absorption and Weight Loss - The water absorption of the PHO films indicated a marked difference between the two aqueous media (Table 1). The percentage of water absorption in the PHO films incubated in water gradually increased with time, reaching 12% and 16% after 12 and 24 months, respectively. In contrast, no significant increase in water absorption was observed in the PHO films incubated in PBS after six months, and the values obtained between 6 and 24 months ranged only between 4 and 5%. The difference here may be attributed to osmotic phenomena and to the ionic strength of the PBS.

The weight loss experienced by the PHO films incubated in water and in isoosmotic PBS was calculated as a percentage of residual weight after 1, 3, 6, 12, and 24 months (Table 1). The weight of the PHO films in both media remained unchanged for the first 6 months. At 12 months, the PHO films incubated in water showed evidence of weight loss (0.5% ± 0.2% s.d.) which slightly progressed to 0.8% ± 0.1% s.d. after 24 months of incubation. The weight loss of the films in PBS was reported in only one PHO film incubated for 24 months.

Mechanical Properties - The mechanical properties of the PHO films were studied by measuring their tensile strength behaviour after incubation in water and in the PBS media (Table 1). The results show that the tensile properties diminished with incubation time, and no significant difference was observed between the two media. A small decrease in breaking strength was observed after one month, remaining constant up to three months. This result may be attributed to the temperature at which the PHO films were incubated because of the low melting temperature of PHO. A gradual reduction in tensile strength was then observed at 6 months, with a 33% and 26% loss for the films incubated in water and in PBS, respectively. Finally, a drastic loss of tensile strength was observed at 24 months in both media, corresponding to a drop of 72% in water and 74% in PBS, as compared to the original tensile strength prior to incubation.

Table 1: Water absorption, weight loss and tensile strength of PHO films incubated in either water or isoosmotic PBS at 37°C for period of 1, 3, 6 and 24 months. Mean (s.d.) n=3.

Conditions	*Time of incubation (months)*	*Water Absorption (%)*	*Weight Loss (%)*	*Tensile Strength (kPa)*
PHO as cast	--	--	--	2.2 (0.2)
	1	3.5 (0.6)	0	1.8 (0.2)
	3	4.5 (1.1)	0	2.0 (0.03)
In water	6	8.2 (4.2)	0.28 (0.15)	1.5 (0.05)
pH 7.0	12	11.1 (2.0)	0.46 (0.21)	1.5 (0.2)
	24	14.6 (3.1)	0.74 (0.05)	0.42 (0.01)
	1	2.6 (1.1)	0	2.1 (0.04)
	3	3.0 (0.3)	0	1.9 (0.06)
In PBS	6	4.7 (2.5)	0	1.6 (0.09)
0.13M pH 7.4	12	4.2 (0.6)	0	1.4 (0.01)
	24	5.1 (1.0)	0.98	0.37 (0.01)

Infrared Spectroscopy - The PHO spectra before incubation showed the typical peaks for the aliphatic C-CH_3 stretchings between 3000 and 2800 cm^{-1} assigned to the alkyl chain of PHO, a strong peak at 1725 cm^{-1} assigned to the carbonyl stretching group, an aliphatic -CH_2- bending band at 1467 cm^{-1}, a C-CH_3 bending at 1380 cm^{-1}, strong peaks of ether C-O stretching in the ester groups at 1320, 1160, and 1100 cm^{-1}, respectively, and a skeletal vibration of $(CH_2)_4$- at 724 cm^{-1}. No chemical changes in terms of shift, height or broadening of the original bands, and no appearance of new peaks in the spectra were observed in the PHO films incubated in either water or PBS for 12 months. However, after 24 months of incubation, significant structural changes in the PHO were detected, as the vibration characteristic of stretching O-H (3200-3600 cm^{-1}) of the hydroxyl group slightly increased. This increase was greater in intensity for the films incubated in PBS, which may be explained by the increased proportion of the hydroxyl groups at both alcohol and carboxylic ends of the polymer chains. Another significant modification of the PHO films incubated in water and in PBS for 24 months was observed in the region ranging between 987 and 970 cm^{-1}. At these peak frequencies, an increase in both the height and the broadening of the peaks was detected. The assignments of these two vibrational frequencies are unknown.

DSC - Measurements of the average glass transition (Tg) and melting (Tm) temperatures as well as the heat of fusion (ΔH) were sequentially obtained by a thermal analysis of the PHO films incubated in water and in isoosmotic PBS for the 24-month incubation period (Table 2). Results show that the Tm of the PHO before incubation (51.4°C) moved to higher temperatures of 55.1 and 54.6°C after one month of incubation in water and in PBS, respectively. In the first 12 months, the Tm did not vary in both media, however, a significant decrease was observed at 24 months, with a Tm value recorded near 48°C. In contrast, the heat of fusion was found to gradually increase in the first 12 months with values ranging between 22.7 and 23.1 J/g at one month and close to 27.5 J/g at 12 months. No significant difference was observed between the aqueous media at each incubation time. While the ΔH of the PHO films incubated in PBS (27.2 J/g ± 0.5 s.d.) remained constant at 24 months, the ΔH of the ones in water decreased to 25.8 J/g ± 1.4 s.d.

Table 2: DSC results of the PHO films incubated in either water or isoosmatic PBS at 37°C for periods of 1, 3, 6, 12 and 24 months. Mean (s.d.) n=3.

Conditions	*Time of incubation (months)*	*Tg (°C)*	*Tm (°C)*	*ΔH (J/g)*
PHO as cast	-	-38.6 (0.3)	51.4 (0.7)	21.9 (2.6)
	1	-37.7 (0.6)	55.1 (0.6)	23.1 (0.1)
	3	-37.5 (0.3)	54.0 (0.2)	24.8 (0.8)
In water	6	-37.7 (0.2)	55.6 (0.2)	25.8 (0.4)
pH 7.0	12	-37.6 (0.8)	55.1 (0.1)	27.4 (0.3)
	24	-39.6 (0.4)	48.7 (0.2)	25.8 (1.4)
	1	-37.7 (0.2)	54.6 (0.8)	22.7 (0.3)
In PBS	3	-37.6 (0.6)	54.6 (0.4)	24.2 (0.1)
0.13M pH 7.4	6	-37.6 (0.3)	55.7 (0.4)	26.5 (0.4)
	12	-39.2 (0.7)	55.0 (0.5)	27.5 (0.3)
	24	-36.9 (0.2)	48.6 (0.2)	27.2 (0.5)

Molecular Weight Measurements - Table 3 shows the percentages of the initial weight average ($\overline{M}$w) and number average ($\overline{M}$n) molecular weight of the PHO films incubated in water or in isoosmotic PBS for 24 months. These results demonstrate that the $\overline{M}$w and the $\overline{M}$n of the PHO both slowly decreased with incubation time, reaching approximately 30% of the initial molecular weight after 24 months of incubation. For the first 12 months, molecular weight loss was significantly faster in the PHO films incubated in PBS than in those incubated in water. However, the PHO films incubated in both media reached similar residual $\overline{M}$w and $\overline{M}$n after 24 months of incubation.

Table 3 : SEC results of the PHO films incubated in either water or isoosmotic PBS at 37°C for periods of 1, 3, 6, 12 and 24 months. Mean (s.d.) n=3.

Conditions	*Time of incubation (months)*	$\overline{M}$ *w (X 10^{-3})*	$\overline{M}$ *n (X 10^{-3})*
PHO as cast	-	119.9 (6.0)	90.6 (7.4)
	1	113.7 (3.6)	78.3 (7.6)
	3	108.1 (3.7)	73.1 (8.9)
Water	6	92.7 (11.8)	68.3 (15.2)
pH 7.0	12	69.1 (4.8)	55.5 (5.0)
	24	32.1 (3.5)	27.1 (3.2)
	1	112.5 (8.2)	82.4 (7.8)
	3	92.9 (4.9)	54.8 (6.4)
PBS	6	52.0 (1.4)	42.1 (3.6)
0.13 M, pH 7.4	12	53.2 (2.0)	38.9 (3.9)
	24	28.2 (3.7)	22.7 (5.0)

In Vivo Biocompatibility and Degradation Studies

Alkaline Phosphatase Secretion (Acute Inflammatory Phase) - The results of the alkaline phosphatase secretion in the tissue/graft specimens are expressed as a ratio of the enzyme secreted for each prosthesis over that of the control (sham-operated) group. These calculations minimized or eliminated the enzyme secretion effect which occurred during the wound repair process following surgery. Figure 2 illustrates that the EO and γ-sterilized PHO grafts induced an intense acute inflammatory reaction after 2 days of implantation, showing ratios of 3.72 ± 0.9 and 3.14 ± 1.0, respectively. These values were not statistically significant when compared to the values of the Dacron® (p=0.02) grafts. On the other hand, the acute response occurred later, and at seven days for the Dacron® graft, which exhibited a milder reaction with a ratio of 1.88 ± 0.94 (ns). The alkaline phosphatase secretion for both PHO grafts was low for the remaining periods of implantation, except for the gamma-sterilized PHO grafts at 30 and 60 days, an increase in enzyme activity of 1.56 ± 0.69 (p=0.03) and 2.20 ± 0.98 (ns), respectively, was recorded. This increase may correspond to inflammatory cell reactivation during the healing sequence.

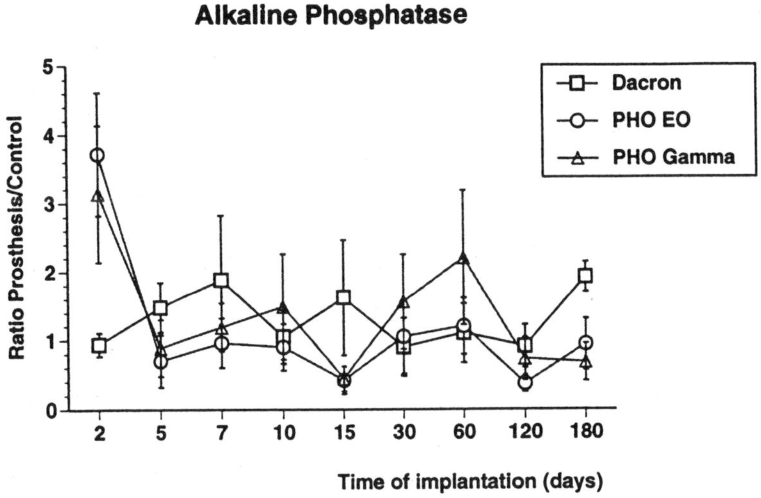

Figure 2 : Alkaline phosphatase activity in the tissue surrounding the Dacron, EO and gamma-sterilized PHO impregnated grafts after implantation. Mean (s.d) n=4.

Acid Phosphatase (Chronic Inflammatory Phase) - Figure 3 presents the results of the acid phosphatase secretion in the tissue/graft specimens which were also calculated as a ratio prosthesis/control. Secretion of acid phosphatase was early for the Dacron® grafts with a ratio at 5 days of 1.94 ± 0.95. Therefore the Dacron® prostheses exhibited a mild chronic inflammatory response up to 180 days of implantation. The onset of chronic inflammation occurred at approximately seven days for the EO and γ-sterilized PHO grafts, with the latter recording the most significant level of intensity with a ratio of 3.21 ± 0.60, compared to 1.72 ± 0.60 for the EO-sterilized PHO graft (p=0.038). For the remaining periods of implantation, these grafts exhibited low acid phosphatase secretion and subsequent mild chronic inflammatory response.

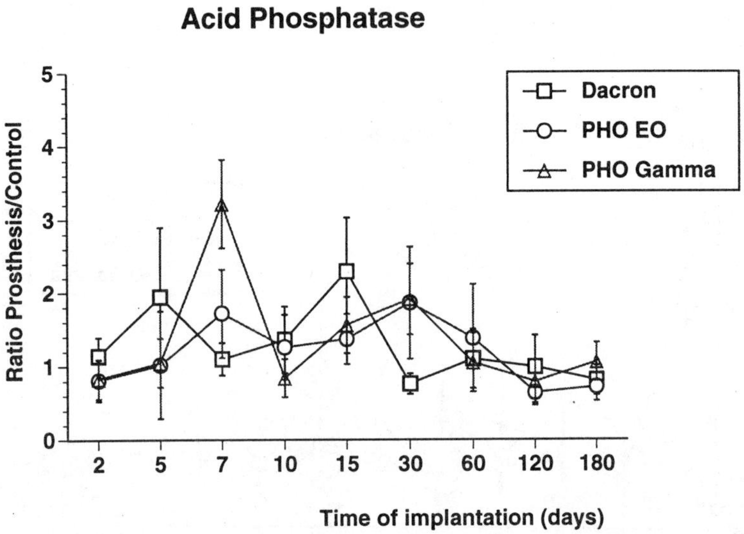

Figure 3 : Acid phosphatase activity in the tissue surrounding the Dacron, EO and gamma-sterilized PHO impregnated grafts after implantation. Mean (s.d.) n=4.

Histological Study - Histological examination of the polyester Dacron® prostheses revealed that a discrete acute inflammatory phase occurred early, at two and five days as a few polymorphonuclear (PMN) cells and lymphocytes were observed near the grafts. This response reached a peak at 7 days with the appearance of numerous PMN cells and lymphocytes. The inflammatory reaction progressed from acute to chronic between 10 and 15 days, and a moderate reaction with macrophages and foreign-body giant cells (FBGCs) was noted. At 15 days, the grafts were filled with a dense fibrin network; however, collagen development was observed externally with some infiltration into the graft wall. The collagen deposition and neovascularization gradually increased between 30 and 120 days, filling the graft wall entirely by day 120. A thick external capsule surrounded the material, and loose, collagenous, fatty tissue was observed inside the prosthetic tube. The level of intensity of the chronic inflammatory reaction decreased with time from a mild reaction at 30 days to a more discrete response at 180 days.

The light microscopic study of the EO and γ-sterilized PHO-impregnated grafts revealed that the healing sequence was similar for both types of grafts. It was demonstrated very early (at two days), that the acute phase was underway, as numerous PMNs cells and lymphocytes had invaded the highly fibrinated implantation site. During the transition phase, which occurred in all of the grafts (between 10 and 15 days), the level of intensity of the reaction had considerably decreased, and a thin collagenous capsule was observed penetrating the graft externally at 15 days. However, this infiltration was limited to approximately 25% of the graft wall thickness for the remaining periods of implantation, with the PHO still present in the graft core. Nevertheless, the chronic inflammatory reaction was generally mild to discrete during this period, except in the γ-sterilized PHO graft at 30 and 60 days, where it increased in its intensity, therefore corroborating the enzymatic study. It was also observed at four and six months post-implantation that the Dacron® polyester fibres impregnated with PHO were separated, either individually or as a bundle from the prosthetic structure, and were isolated by inflammatory cells and collagenous tissue.

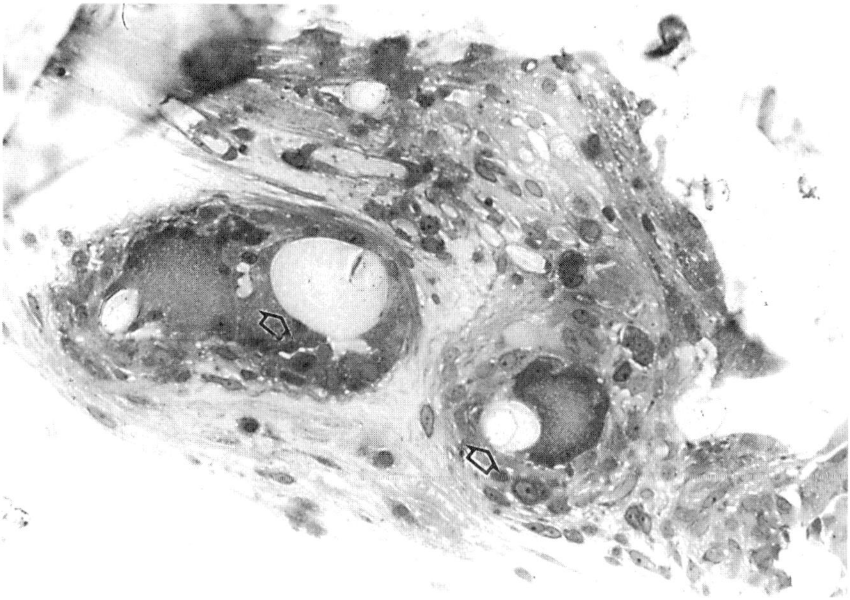

Figure 4 : Light photomicrograph of the EO-sterilized PHO graft after 4 months of implantation in rats (X 400).

Figure 4 presents this phenomenon, and suggests that Dacron® fibres and PHO were fragmented by an enzymatic attack. The reaction was driven by macrophages and by FBGCs which were observed engulfing individual Dacron® fibres with PHO into cytoplasmic extension (arrows). After 6 months of implantation, tissue development remained limited to the external part of the graft (EC) with some areas of collagen infiltration in between multifilament yarns (arrows) (Figure 5). These areas of tissue penetration may be the result of the PHO degradation by enzymes or the inconsistant or irregular impregnation of PHO during graft preparation. Finally, PHO was mostly present in the graft core after 6 months of implantation and consequently will require substantial hydrolytic scission of the ester bonds into low molecular weight oligomers before any bioresorption phenomenon can be observed *in vivo*.

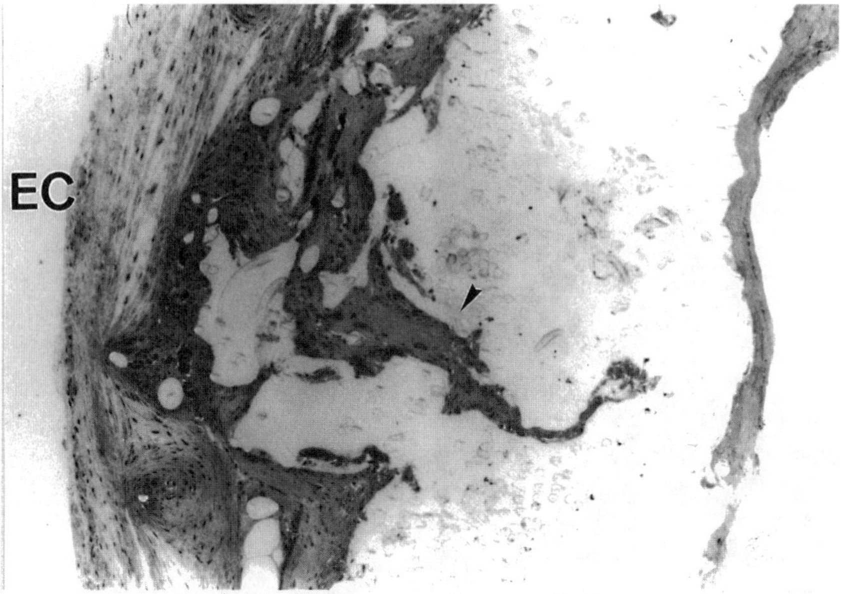

Figure 5 : Light photomicrograph of the EO-sterilized PHO graft after 6 months of implantation in rats (X 100).

DSC Study - The average melting (Tm) temperature and heat of fusion (ΔH) obtained from thermal analyses of the EO and γ-sterilized PHO grafts after implantation as shown in Table 4. Results show that the gamma radiation sterilization reduced the Tm from 58.5°C to 55.2°C, while the Tm after EO sterilization remained unchanged at 58.5°C. Upon implantation, the Tm and ΔH of the γ-sterilized PHO were both significantly reduced to 52.7°C ($p=0.008$) and 9.4 J/g ($p=0.001$) respectively, while only a slight decrease was observed in the Tm and ΔH of the EO-sterilized PHO grafts (ns). For the remaining periods of implantation, the Tm of the EO-sterilized PHO showed no significant variation, whereas a gradual increase in the heat of fusion was observed with time, reaching a value of 17.0 ± 1.2 J/g at 180 days of implantation ($p=0.031$). The Tm of the γ-sterilized PHO ranged between 52.7°C ± 0.5 at 2 days and 53.3 ± 0.02°C at 15 days, although a significant increase occurred at 30 days with a value of 55°C ($p=0.004$), i.e., that of the Tm after gamma sterilization. A similar pattern of events also occurred with the heat of fusion. Up to 15 days, the ΔH of the γ-sterilized PHO was approximately 9 J/g. However, a significant increase in ΔH was observed at 30 days with a value of 15.4 ± 1.2 J/g ($p=0.042$) which remained stable thereafter with time, reaching 16.0 ± 1.1 J/g after 180 days of implantation.

Table 4: DSC results of the PHO grafts implanted subcutaneously in rats for periods ranging between 2 and 180 days. Mean (s.d.) n=4.

Prostheses	*Duration of implantation (days)*	*Tm (°C)*	*ΔH (J/g)*
EO-PHO grafts	0	58.5 (0)	13.1 (0)
	2	57.1 (0)	11.8 (0)
	5	59.5 (0.5)	14.8 (1.4)
	7	59.4 (0.1)	14.3 (0.7)
	10	57.7 (0.8)	13.1 (0.2)
	15	59.5 (0.4)	14.5 (0.5)
	30	58.5 (0.9)	15.1 (1.3)
	60	56.6 (0.3)	14.7 (1.4)
	120	57.0 (0.6)	15.8 (0.6)
	180	58.2 (0.9)	17.0 (1.2)
Gamma-PHO grafts	0	55.2 (0)	13.0 (0)
	2	52.7 (0.5)	9.4 (0)
	5	54.2 (2.3)	8.6 (1.3)
	7	54.3 (0)	8.0 (0)
	10	53.1 (0.9)	7.9 (1.4)
	15	53.3 (0.1)	9.5 (0.8)
	30	55.5 (0.1)	15.4 (1.2)
	60	55.1 (0.7)	15.1 (0.4)
	120	55.1 (1.1)	15.3 (0.7)
	180	55.9 (0.5)	16.0 (1.1)

Molecular Weight Measurements - The changes in both weight average ($\overline{M}$w) and number average ($\overline{M}$n) molecular weight of the PHO were measured both before and after sterilization as well as after 1, 2, 4 and 6 months of implantation in the rat. Figure 6 shows that the $\overline{M}$w of the γ-sterilized PHO decreased after sterilization by 16.6% ± 1.8% (p=0.004) while that of the EO-sterilized graft slightly decreased only (4.7% ± 0.4 %). Upon implantation, the $\overline{M}$w of the EO and γ-sterilized PHO gradually decreased by 29.1% ± 1.1% and 22.7% ± 1.6% respectively after six months of implantation as compared to the value on day 0 (p=0.001). The results observed with the $\overline{M}$n also showed the same trend as with the $\overline{M}$w. A decrease in $\overline{M}$n of 25.5% ± 2.7% (p=0.005) was observed after gamma sterilization, which was more significant than that following EO sterilization (5.2%). Compared to the $\overline{M}$n on day 0, the $\overline{M}$n of the EO and γ-sterilized PHO decreased in a similar fashion, showing a reduction of 27.9% ± 3.0% and 19.8% ± 4.5, respectively (p=0.001). Throughout this study, the polydispersity of the EO and γ-sterilized PHO remained unchanged after sterilization as well as after implantation.

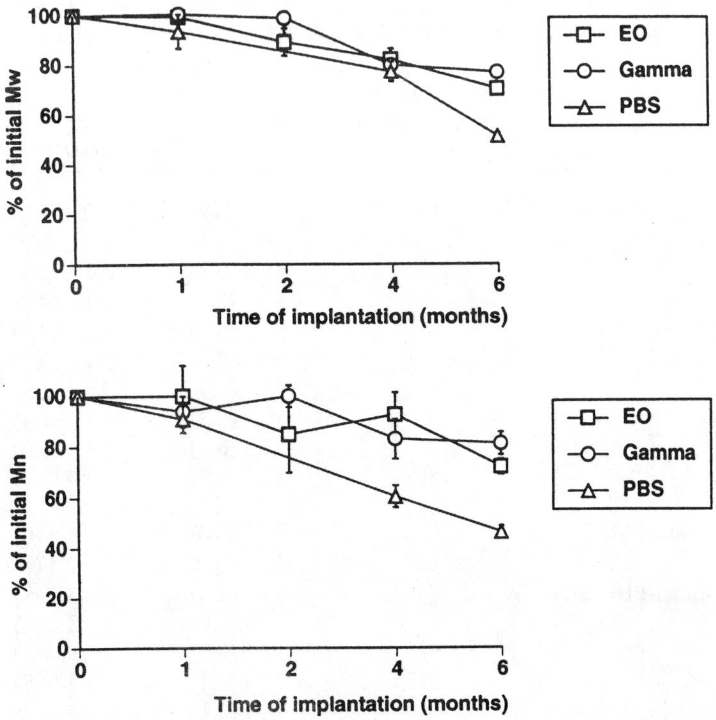

Figure 6 : SEC results of the EO and gamma-sterilized PHO implanted subcutaneously in rats. Results of the PHO incubated in PBS is added for comparison.

In Vivo Healing Behaviour of PHO-Impregnated Grafts

Implantations and Follow- up - All eight implantations were uneventful without any morbidity or mortality. The time needed to perform the anastomoses of the preclotted PET grafts and PHO impregnated grafts was 42.5 ± 19.1 min and 44.0 ±15.3 min respectively. The handling and suturing characteristics of the preclotted grafts were excellent while PHO impregnated grafts demonstrated graft stiffness and hardness during needle insertion. After restoration of the blood flow, there was minimal bleeding through the anastomotic lines for both grafts and the PHO impregnated grafts were completely impervious to blood.

Macroscopic Observations and Patency

All preclotted and PHO impregnated prostheses were patent after one month of implantation. The luminal surface of all the preclotted polyester grafts was covered by a thin thrombotic matrix. The anastomotic regions of three out of four preclotted grafts were white and glistening. In contrast, two PHO impregnated grafts showed a thick thrombotic matrix laying over the entire graft while the last two were covered by isolated small thrombi and exhibiting white and glistening surfaces. Externally, all the preclotted and PHO impregnated grafts were incorporated by a thick collagenous tissue and there was no evidence of peripheric mural hematoma.

Histological and Scanning Electron Microscopy

Preclotted PET grafts : Histological observation of the preclotted PET grafts revealed that three out of four prostheses were fairly incorporated by healing tissue. Both proximal and distal regions of the grafts were covered by a thin collagenous capsule (IC) which infiltrated the porous structure (Figure 7). This tissue lining was covered by endothelial-like cells as revealed by scanning electron micrographs. The healing in the medial region was characterized by mixed areas of thrombus and reorganized matrix by collagenous tissue. The luminal surface of the fourth preclotted graft showed thrombotic deposits over the entire length with evidence of reorganized collagenous matrix distally. All of the grafts were externally encapsulated by a thick collagenous tissue (EC) and the graft wall demonstrated a moderate chronic inflammatory response with numerous macrophages and a few FBGC.

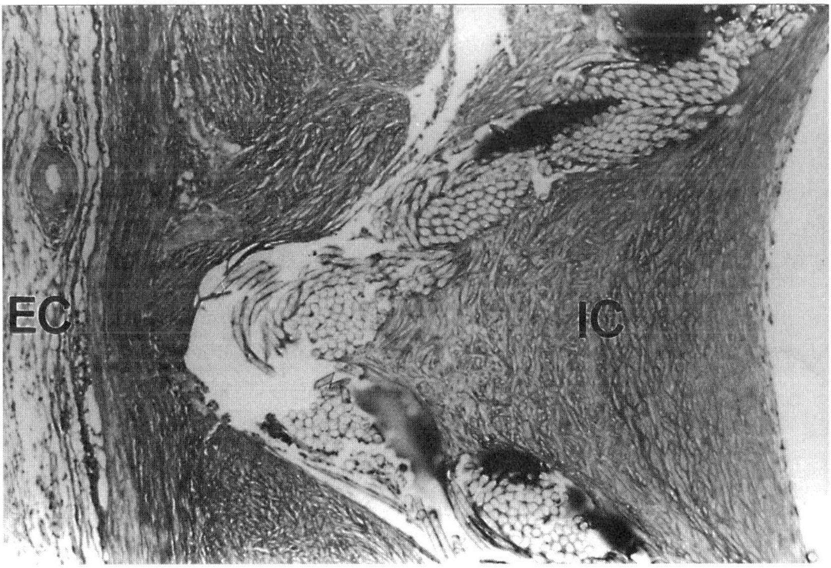

Figure 7 : Light photomicrograph of a cross-section of the proximal region of the preclotted Dacron arterial prosthesis after one month of implantation in dogs (X 100).

PHO Impregnated Grafts – Light microscopic examination of the luminal surface of the PHO impregnated grafts revealed that two PHO grafts showed satisfactory healing sequence characterized by the development of a thin collagenous internal capsule (IC) and endothelial cell coverage. The collagenous tissue was seen infiltrating the innermost portion of the graft between the yarns (Figure 8). The infiltration of collagen was less than that observed with the preclotted grafts. For the other grafts, the proximal region showed a beginning of collagenous capsule development internally while the internal capsule was more complete in the distal region with the evidence of endothelial-like cells. Medially, the luminal surface was covered by a thrombotic matrix in reorganization with occasional islets of endothelial-like cells. A thicker collagenous tissue surrounded the external portion of the grafts (EC) which was associated with a moderate chronic inflammatory reaction.

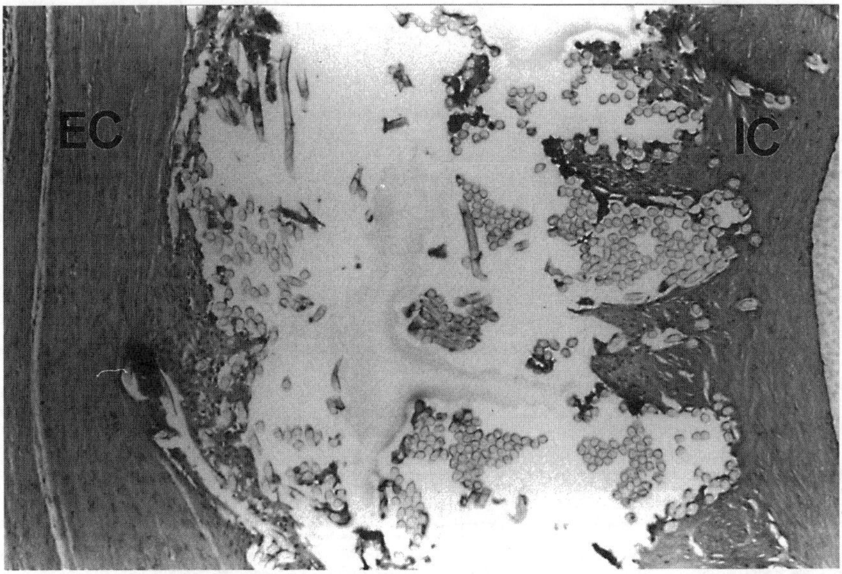

Figure 8 : Light photomicrograph of a cross-section of the proximal region of the EO sterilized PHO impregnated graft after one month of implantation in dogs (X 100).

Prostacyclin / Thromboxane A_2 Secretion Study

Figure 9 shows the mean PGI_2/TXA_2 ratios of the proximal, medial and distal regions of the preclotted and PHO impregnated grafts after one month of implantation. The mean PGI_2/TXA_2 ratios of the proximal area of the preclotted and PHO impregnated grafts were 3.6 ± 0.4 and 1.3 ± 0.4, respectively and the difference was statistically significant by one way ANOVA analysis ($p = 0.01$). In the medial region, the PGI_2/TXA_2 secretion of the PET graft (1.0 ± 0.7) was higher than that of the PHO impregnated grafts (0.5 ± 0.1). No significant difference was detected by ANOVA. Distally, the preclotted grafts demonstrated a greater PGI_2/ TXA_2 ratio (1.9 ± 1.1) than that of the PHO impregnated grafts (0.8 ± 0.4). This result was not significant. The segments of abdominal aorta used as controls exhibited a high PGI_2/ TXA_2 secretion ratio of 22.3 ± 7.8 (n = 8).

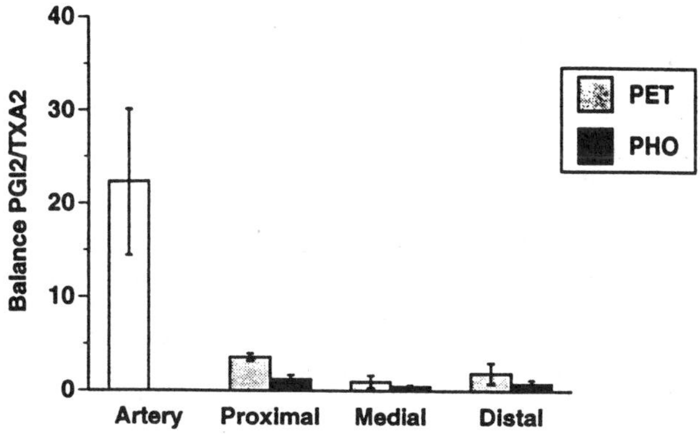

Figure 9 : Prostacyclin (PGI_2) and Thromboxane (TXA_2) secretion by the luminal surfaces of the preclotted and PHO impregnated grafts after one month of implantation.

Discussion

The present investigation was undertaken to assess the sterilization, degradation rate and biocompatibility of a bacterial polyester polyhydroxyoctanoate as a potential sealant for the polyester arterial prosthesis. The discussion which follows will examine the various physical and structural changes occurring after the sterilization of PHO, describe the mechanism and rate of degradation of PHO both in vitro and in vivo, and address the biocompatibility of PHO and its potential use for vascular surgery applications.

Effects of Sterilization

This study concerned two common sterilization techniques used for medical devices, namely, EO gas and gamma radiation. Ethylene oxide gas is a very effective, highly diffusive bactericide which can be used at temperatures below 60°C. Its bacterial properties depend on exposure time, temperature, and moisture. The only drawback is the toxicity of residual amounts trapped in the device which can be overcome by sufficient aeration. As an alternative to EO gas, gamma radiation is a simple and highly penetrating method involving only one variable, namely, exposure time. However, the effects of this ionizing radiation on polymers may result in alterations to the molecular structure of the polymer, such as the formation of nonmetabolized or non-excreted products which may affect the biocompatibility and bioresorption rate of the polymer. Two major phenomena have been described. The first is a degradation mechanism, which occurs by a random chain scission of chemical bonds and a subsequent reduction in the molecular weight of the polymer. The second is a cross-linking mechanism of polymer molecules, which results in the formation of three-dimensional networks.

Investigation of the bulk chemistry of PHO revealed that gamma radiation induced a significant reduction of $\overline{M}$w and $\overline{M}$*n*, whereas no significant decrease in molecular weight was observed following EO sterilization. This phenomenon has been reported elsewhere with several degradable polymers *[8-12]*. The DSC results also revealed that the Tm and heat of fusion of the gamma-sterilization were modified after sterilization. The Tm was shown to have slightly decreased, which may be attributed to the decrease in the molecular weight or chain scission. On the other hand, the increase in the heat of fusion may be explained by a predominant and selective random scission occurring in the amorphous region and the subsequent formation of crystallites from degraded macromolecular chains formed by chain scission. This process may have enhanced the physical cross-linking effect as shown by the increase of tensile strength experienced by the gamma-sterilized PHO films. It was suggested that polymers containing oxygen in their backbone were exceptionnally susceptible to radiation, and that the quaternary carbon was the atom responsible for the cross-linking reaction *[13]*. De Koning et al. showed that the alkyl pendent chain of medium-chain-length PHAs (such as PHO) was reactive to cross-linking *[14]*. As observed with many irradiated polymers, cross-linking results in an initial increase in tensile strength with a decreased impact strength and a more brittle appearance with increased radiation dose *[15]*.

In a study on the effect of radiation on polyethylene terephthalate, Nair et al. also demonstrated molecular weight loss, increase in the heat of fusion and crystallinity and a slight increase in tensile properties *[16]*. They concluded that degradation, followed by recombination of macromolecular chains in the amorphous region, increased crystallinity and that cross-linking occurred during recombination.

Mechanism and rate of degradation of PHO

Results of the present study demonstrate that the in vitro degradation of PHO in either water or physiologic buffer saline media is a long process which exceeds two years and is governed by a hydrolytic mechanism involving ester bond cleavage of polymer chains with gradual reduction of the $\overline{M}$w and $\overline{M}$n. Other PHAs such as PHB or copolymers PHB/HV and PHB/HB have also shown long-term degradation profiles *[17-20]*. First, the greater liquid absorption in water, as opposed to PBS reported here has also been observed with poly (α-hydroxy acids) *[21-23]* and other biodegradable polymer *[8,24]*. This phenomenon has been attributed to the ionic strength of the PBS aqueous buffer medium *[22]*. The greater $\overline{M}$w and $\overline{M}$n decreases recorded for the PHO films incubated in PBS between 6 and 12 months may be explained by the ionic strength and buffer effect of PBS which accelerates ester bond cleavage. It has been shown that the conversion of acidic degradation products into neutral salts catalyzes hydrolysis, causes more rapid loss of tensile strength *[25]* and is influenced by the salt concentration in the buffer solutions *[26]*. Similar phenomena were observed with other degradable polymers *[22,27]*. On the other hand, the effect of acidic conversion products on the degradation of PHO may be attenuated by the show degradation rate of the polymer. The crystallization of the hydrolized polymer chains may explain the PHO's similar tensile properties observed in the water and PBS conditions.

The significant change in the FTIR spectra of the PHO films incubated in either water or PBS after 24 months of incubation i.e. the observation of increased OH groups, suggest that the process of hydrolysis may have begun internally, moving to the surface of the films. In large-sized specimen, this process of faster internal degradation has been recognized for some time and is associated with water diffusion in the material which progresses toward the surface, at which time a hollow structure remains to be degraded *[28]*. However, a few studies on thin films have shown no faster internal degradation *[28,29]*.

The DSC results confirmed that the degradation of PHO, as with other semi-crystalline polymers, occurs in two stages. First, there is a random hydrolytic scission of ester bonds in the amorphous region which progresses during the first 12 months of incubation as the Tm of the PHO remains constant. During that time, a recombination of the polymer chains may explain the increase in the heat of fusion and possibly, the percentage of crystallinity. Second, the drop of both Tm and ΔH between 12 and 24 months may reflect the hydrolytic attack of the crystalline domain and thus, the second stage of hydrolysis. It is important to note that in the amorphous zone, the hydrolysis into oligomer by-products is not eliminated from the film prior to attacking the remaining crystalline zone because of the size morphology effect of thin films. The fate of oligomer degradation products removed from the film remains to be elucidated.

In vivo studies dealing with biodegradable polymers must determine the mechanism and rate of degradation occurring during implantation by investigating the polymer after retrieval. As shown in vitro, the PHO exhibited a slow biodegradation rate characterized by a gradual reduction of molecular weight typical of a hydrolytic mechanism involving random ester bond cleavage. The DSC results confirmed the preferential scission in the amorphous zone and the recombination of the macromolecular chains that slightly crystallized the copolymer as revealed by the increase in the heat of fusion. Following implantation, the gamma-sterilized PHO experienced an additional decrease in both Tm and ΔH which suggests taht the crystalline zone of PHO is further affected at 37°C. The reason for this remains unclear, however, the instability of the macromolecular chains cleaved in the crystalline structure during gamma radiation may possibly further destabilize after implantation.

Our study also suggests the possible contribution of enzymes in the degradation of PHO, albeit to a lesser extent than the hydrolytic process. Enzymes secreted by inflammatory cells such as macrophages and FBGC may participate in the degradation process by isolating fragments of polymer, a phenomenon observed histologically. However, most of the polymer will be submitted to an hydrolytic process characterized by the gradual formation of low molecular fragments at which time, the enzymes may easily be involved as the final contributor to the degradation. For the PHO, this process may require several months, possibly years in vivo, before complete disappearance of the polymer can be observed. Of note, a recent study revealed that a PHB patch implanted in the pericardium of humans was still observed 24 months after implantation *[30]*.

Biocompatibility and healing behaviour of PHO as a sealant for arterial prosthesis

The present investigation on PHO revealed that PHO is biocompatible, as no adverse inflammatory reactions occurred after implantation in rats or dogs. Indeed, following a strong, early acute reaction, as revealed by the enzymatic study, the inflammatory reaction quickly progressed to a chronic response of relatively low intensity as seen with the Dacron prosthesis for the remaining periods of implantation. The greater inflammatory response observed with gamma-sterilized PHO grafts as compared to EO-sterilized PHO grafts is not surprising, as other investigators have also reported on the adverse effects of radiation sterilization on the physico-chemical and biological properties of macromolecules and polymer biomaterials *[31,32]*.

As an infrarenal aortic substitute in dogs, the EO-sterilized PHO impregnated graft was impervious to blood but its handling and suturing characteristics need to be optimized to obtain a more pliable graft with lower prosthetic drag properties. This will be achieved by optimizing the amount of PHO impregnated in the porous polyester structure. The healing sequence of the PHO impregnated prosthesis was slightly delayed as compared to the preclotted graft. While two PHO grafts were covered by thrombotic deposits, two showed evidence of healing characterized by internal collagenous capsule development at both anastomotic sites, progressing toward the mid-portion of the graft and by endothelialization as revealed by histological and SEM studies as well as PGI_2/TXA_2 secretion measurements. This delay in the healing of PHO impregnated prosthesis is caused by the slow bioresorption rate of the copolymer although its presence does not impair the capacity of the graft to heal. The PHO is still present in the graft skeleton after one month of implantation and there is evidence of external collagenous tissue development, infiltration and incorporation into the graft wall contributing to the stabilization of the prosthetic structure. Interestingly, when compared to other widely used and commercially available protein impregnated grafts, the PHO graft exhibited similar healing characteristics in terms of PGI_2 /TXA_2 secretion to that of a gelatin impregnated graft *[33]*, and greater PGI_2 /TXA_2 ratio than those observed with a carbodiimide cross-linked gelatin *[34]* and a glutaraldehyde cross-linked albumin *[35]*.

Because protein impregnated grafts promote undesirable immunological reaction caused by the xenogenic nature of the substrate or the release of cross-linking molecules, and because they are under scrutiny by regulatory agencies, new biological or synthetic substrate that are biodegradable and most of all non-antigenic so as to limit the inflammatory response must be developed. As an alternative to protein impregnated grafts, PHO is one potential sealant for the polyester arterial prosthesis whose preliminary in vivo behaviour has shown satisfactory healing characteristics. Further investigations will aim at optimizing the amount of PHO to be impregnated in polyester knitted arterial prostheses with regard to imperviousness and promoting a fast and complete healing sequence on the luminal surface.

Acknowledgments

This study was supported by the Québec Biomaterials Institute. We are indebted to Valerie Bélanger, Suzanne Bourassa, Martin Castonguay, Claire Kingston, Claude-Paul Lafrance, Claire Letendre and Aristide Pusterla (Microscopy Service, RSVS, Laval University) for their technical assistance. We also thank Rodica Plesu and Dr. Robert E. Prud'homme for kindly providing us access to SEC and X-ray instruments.

References

[*1*] Anderson, A.J., Dawes, E.A., "Occurrence, Metabolism, Metabolic Role, and Industrial Uses of Bacterial Polyhydroxyalkanoates", Microbiol. Rev., Vol. 24, 1990, pp. 450-472.

[*2*] Malm, T., Bowald, S., Bylock, A., Busch, C., Saldeen, T., "Enlargement of the Right Ventricular Outflow Tract and the Pulmonary Artery with a New Biodegradable Patch in Transannular Position", Eur. Surg. Res., Vol. 26, 1994, pp. 298-308.

[*3*] Malm, T., Bowald, S., Bylock, A., Saldeen, T., Busch, C., "Regeneration of Pericardial Tissue on Absorbable Polymer Patches Implanted into the Pericardial Sac", Scand. J. Thor. Cardiovasc. Surg., Vol. 26, 1992, pp. 15-21.

[*4*] Kostopoulos, L., Karring, T., "Guided Bone Regeneration in Mandibular Defects in Rats Using a Bioresorbable Polymer", Clin. Oral Impl. Res., Vol. 5, 1994, pp. 66-74.

[*5*] Gross, R.A, DeMello, C., Lenz, R.W., Fuller, R.C., "Biosynthesis and Characterization of Poly(β-hydroxyalkanoates) Produced by *Pseudomonas oleovorans*", Macromolecules, Vol. 22, 1989, pp. 1106-1115.

[6] Standard Specification for Tensile Testing Machines for Textiles, ASTM D-7693, Annual Book of ASTM Standards, Vol. 07.01, American Society for Testing and Materials, Philadelphia, PA 1993.

[7] Schakenraad, J.M., Nieuwenhuis, P., Molenaar, I., Helder, J., Dijkstra P.J., Feijen, J., *In vivo* and *in vitro* degradation of glycine / DL-lactic acid copolymers, J. Biomed. Mater. Res., 1989; 23 : 1271.

[8] Ertel, S.I., Kohn, J., "Evaluation of a Series of Tyrosine-Derived Polycarbonates as Degradable Biomaterials, J. Biomed. Mater. Res., Vol. 28, 1994, pp. 919-930.

[9] Spenlehauer, G., Vert, M., Benoit, J.P., Boddaert, A., "*In Vitro* and I*n Vivo* Degradation of Poly (D,L lactide / glycolide) Type Microspheres Made by Solvent Evaporation Method", Biomaterials, Vol. 10, 1989, pp. 557-563.

[*10*] Volland, C., Wolff, M., Kissel, T., "The Influence of Terminal Gamma-Sterilization on Captopril Containing Poly (D, L -lactide-co-glycolide) Microspheres", J. Controlled Release, Vol. 31, 1994, pp. 293-305.

[*11*] Claes, L.E., Ignatius, A.A., Rehm, K.E., Scholz, C., "New Bioresorbable Pin for the Reduction of Small Bony Fragments: Design, Mechanical Properties, and *In vitro* Degradation", Biomaterials, Vol. 17, 1996, pp. 1621-1626.

[*12*] Merkli, A., Heller, J., Tabataboy, C., Murray, R., "Gamma Sterilization of a Semi-Solid Poly(ortho ester) Designed for Controlled Drug Delivery. Validation and Radiation Effects", Pharm. Res., Vol. 11, 1994, pp. 1485-1491.

[*13*] Gupta, M.C., Deshmukh, V.G., "Radiation Effects on Poly (lactic acid)", Polymer, Vol. 24, 1983, pp. 827-830.

[*14*] De Koning, G.J.M., van Bilsen, H.M.M., Lemstra, P.J., Hazenberg, W., Witholt, B., Preusting, H., van der Galien, J.G., Schirmer, A., Jendrossek, D., "A Biodegradable Rubber by Cross-Linking Poly(hydroxyalkanoate) from *Pseudomonas oleovorans* ", Polymer, Vol. 35, 1994, pp. 2090-2097.

[*15*] Dempsey, D.J., Thirucote, R.R., "Sterilization of Medical Devices: A review", J. Biomat. Appl., Vol. 3, 1989, pp. 454-523.

[*16*] Nair, P.D., Sreenivasan, K., Jayabalan, M., "Multiple Gamma Radiation Sterilization of Polyester Fibres", Biomaterials, Vol. 9, 1988, pp. 335-338.

[*17*] Doi, Y., Kanesawa, Y., Kawaguchi, Y., Kunioka, M., "Hydrolytic Degradation of Microbial Poly(hydroxyalkanoates)", Makromol. Chem., Rapid Commun., Vol. 10, 1989, pp. 227-230.

[*18*] Kunioka, M., Kawaguchi, Y., Doi, Y., "Production of Biodegradable Copolyesters of 3-hydroxybutyrate and 4-hydroxybutyrate by *Alcaligenes eutrophus*", Appl. Microbiol. Biotechnol., Vol. 30, 1989, pp. 569-573.

[*19*] Knowles, J.C., "Development of a Natural Degradable Polymer for Orthopaedic Use", J. Med. Eng. Tech., Vol. 17, 1993, pp. 129-137.

[20] Brandl, H., Bachofen, R., Mayer, J., Wintermantel, E., "Degradation and Applications of Polyhydroxyalkanoates, Can. J. Microbiol., Vol. 41, 1995, pp. 143-153.

[21] Li, S.M., Garreau, H., Vert, M., "Structure-Property Relationships in the Case of the Degradation of Massive Aliphatic Poly-(α-hydroxyacids) in Aqueous Media. Part 1: Poly (DL-lactic acid)", J. Mater. Sci., Materials in Medicine, Vol. 1, 1990, pp. 123-130.

[22] Li, S.M., Garreau, H., Vert, M., "Structure Property Relationships in the Case of the Degradation of Massive Aliphatic Poly- (α-hydroxyacids) in Aqueous Media. Part 2 : Degradation of Lactic-acid-glycolide copolymers : PLA37.5 GA25 and PLA75 GA25", J. Mater. Sci., Materials in Medicine, Vol. 1, 1990, pp. 131-139.

[*23*] Li SM, Garreau H, Vert M. "Structure-Property Relationships in the Case of the Degradation of Massive Aliphatic Poly-(α-hydroxyacids) in Aqueous Media. Part 3: Influence of the Morphology of Poly-(L-lactic acid) ", J. Mater. Sci.: Materials in Medicine, Vol. 1, 1990, pp. 198-206.

[*24*] Richards, M., Dahiyat, B.I., Arm, D.M., Brown, P.R, Leong, K.W., "Evaluation of Polyphosphates and Polyphosphonates as Degradable Biomaterials", J. Biomed. Mater. Res., Vol. 25, 1991, pp. 1151-1167.

[*25*] Chu, C.C., "An In Vitro Study of the Effect of Buffer on the Degradation of Poly(glycolic acid) Sutures", J. Biomed. Mater. Res., Vol. 15, 1981, pp. 19-27.

[*26*] Makino, K., Ohshima, H., Kondo, T., "Mechanism of Hydrolytic Degradation of Poly(L-lactide) Microcapsules: Effects of pH, Ionic Strength and Buffer Concentration", J. Microencapsulation, Vol. 3, 1986, pp. 203-212.

[*27*] Bueno Martinez, M., Molina Pinilla, I., Zamora Mata, F., Galbis Pérez JA., "Hydrolytic Degradation of Poly(ester amides) Derived from Carbohydrates", Macromolecules, Vol. 30, 1997, pp. 3197-3203.

[*28*] Li, S.M., Vert, M., "Biodegradation of Aliphatic Polyesters. In: "Degradable Polymers; Principles and Applications", G. Scott and D. Gilead (eds.), Chapman and Hall Publishers, London, UK, 1995, pp. 43-87.

[*29*] Mauduit, J., Pérouse, E., Vert, M., "Hydrolytic Degradation of Films Prepared from Blends of High and Low Molecular Weight Poly (DL-lactic acids)", J. Biomed. Mater. Res., Vol. 30, 1990, pp. 201-207.

[*30*] Duvernoy, O., Malm, T., Ramstrom, J., Bowald, S., "A Biodegradable Patch Used as a Pericardial Substitute after Cardiac Surgery: 6- and 24-Month Evaluation with CT", Thorac. Cardiovasc. Surgeon, Vol. 43, 1995 pp. 271-274.

[*31*] Bruck, S.D., Meller, E.P., "Radiation Sterilization of Polymeric Implant Materials", J. Biomed. Mater. Res., Vol. 22, Suppl. A2, 1988, pp. 133-144.

[*32*] Cheung, D.T., Peselman, N., Tong, D., Nimmi, M.E., "The Effect of Gamma-Irradiation on Collagen Molecules, Isolated Alpha-Chains and Cross-Linked Native Fibres". J. Biomed. Mater. Res., Vol. 24, 1990, pp. 581-589.

[*33*] Chafké, N., Marois, Y., Guidoin, R., Deng, X., Marois, M., Roy, R., King, M., Douville, Y., "Biocompatibility and Biofunctionality of a Gelatin Impregnated Polyester Arterial Prosthesis". Polymers & Polymer Composites, Vol. 4, 1993, pp. 229-251.

[*34*] Marois, Y., Chafké, N., Deng, X., Marois, M., How T., King M., Guidoin R., "Carbodiimide Cross-Linked Gelatin : A New Coating for Porous Polyester Arterial Prostheses", Biomaterials, Vol. 16, 1995, pp. 1131-1139.

[*35*] Marois, Y., Chafké, N., Guidoin, R., Duhamel, R.C., Roy, R., Marois, M., King, M., Douville, Y., "An Albumin-Coated Polyester Arterial Graft : In Vivo Assessment of Biocompatibility and Healing Characteristics", Biomaterials, Vol. 17, 1996, pp. 3-14.

Katarzyna Gorna,[1] and Sylwester Gogolewski[2]

Novel Biodegradable Polyurethanes for Medical Applications

Reference: Gorna, K., and Gogolewski, S., **"Novel Biodegradable Polyurethanes for Medical Applications,"** *Synthetic Bioabsorbable Polymers for Implants, ASTM STP 1396,* C. M. Agrawal, J. E. Parr, and S. T. Lin, Eds. American Society for Testing and Materials, West Conshohocken, PA, 2000.

Abstract: Biodegradable polyurethanes with various hydrophilic-to-hydrophobic ratios and potential application for nonadhesive barriers in surgery and/or scaffolds for tissue engineering and bone substitutes were synthesized from polycaprolactone diol, mixtures of polycaprolactone and polyethylene oxide diols, hexamethylene- and/or isophorone diiscocyanates, and 1,4-butane diol or 2-amino-1-butanol chain extenders. The polymers had viscosity-average molecular weights in the range of 24.000 to 130.000 dalton, tensile strengths at break of 4 to 60 MPa, Young's moduli from 7 to 72 MPa, elongation at break of 100 to 950%, and glass transition temperatures in the range of -116 to -41°C. The affinity of polymers towards proteins varied depending on the type of polyol and the chain extender used. The adsorption of proteins from whole blood was highest for the materials based on poly(ε-caprolactone) and those containing 2-amino-1-butanol chain extender. There was no protein adsorption on materials based on mixtures of caprolactone and ethylene oxide polyols independent of the poly(ethylene oxide) molecular weight and the chain extender used. The polymers could be processed into three-dimensional porous scaffolds (membranes and sponges) using a phase-inverse process from solutions consisting of a solvent-nonsolvent system and/or with salt crystals additives.

Keywords: biodegradable materials, polyurethanes, polymer synthesis, protein adsorption, nonadhesive barriers, porous scaffolds

For years, polyurethane elastomers have been used in intracorporeal and extracorporeal devices. Pacing leads insulation, indwelling catheters, intra-aortic balloons, total artificial hearts, heart valves, ventricular assist devices, vascular prostheses, vascular stents, and angioplasty balloons are typical examples of cardiovascular applications. Polyurethanes are also used in mammary implants, oesophageal and tracheal prostheses, ureteral prostheses, fallopian tubings, endotracheal tubings, gastric balloons, feeding tubings, catheters, cannulae, dialysis membranes, filters in blood oxygenators, blood bags, wound

[1]Ph.D. Student, Polymer Research, AO/ASIF Research Institute, CH-7270 Davos, Switzerland.
[2]Professor and Head, Polymer Research, AO/ASIF Research Institute, CH-7270 Davos, Switzerland.

dressings, drapes, sutures, ligaments and orthopaedic casting tapes [*1,2*]. Experimentally, they were used in peripheral nerve repair devices, implants for craniofacial and maxillofacial reconstruction, liners in dentistry, paradental membranes, shock absorbing elements for root implants, adhesives, drug delivery devices, enveloping membranes for soft organ fixation, meniscus reconstruction membranes, artificial kidneys, implants for craniofacial and maxillofacial reconstruction are typical examples of such products [*1,2*].

One of the primary concerns with polyurethanes for implantable devices is their molecular stability *in vivo*. The biologically active environment of the living body degrades the majority of medical polyurethanes, mainly through hydrolytic chain scission within ester and urethane linkages of a polymer and oxidative attack within polyether segments, processes which can be facilitated by the presence of enzymes and cell peroxides [*1-5*]. The relative molecular instability of polyurethanes may, however, be deliberately exploited to design biodegradable implants.

In recent years, the efforts have been made to design biodegradable polyurethanes [*6-31*]. This is generally achieved by incorporating labile moieties susceptible to hydrolysis in the polymer chain. Thus, experimental degradable polyurethanes were synthesized in the early eighties by using diols based on copolymers of lactic acid with ethylene diol or diethylene diol [*6*]. This concept was later exploited to obtain degradable polyurethanes from diols based on lactic acid and 1,4-butanediol [*7-11*] and butyric acid and ethylene diol [*12-14*]. Degradable polyurethanes were also obtained from monomers containing peptide links [*15-17*], sugar derivatives [*18-24*], hydroxy-terminated copolymers of L-lactide-ε-caprolactone, glycolide-ε-caprolactone [*25*], ε-caprolactone-co-δ-valerolactone [*26,27*], lysine diisocyanate [*25,28-30*], poly(ethylene oxide), poly(ε-caprolactone) and amino acid-based chain extender [*31*].

Depending on their mechanical properties, chemical composition and surface characteristics, such biodegradable polyurethanes can potentially be used for cardiovascular implants, drug delivery devices, nonadhesive barriers in trauma surgery, cancellous bone graft substitutes, injectable augmentation materials, tissue - organ regeneration scaffolds (tissue engineering), or adhesives. In the early eighties biodegradable polyurethanes based on lactide diols and hexamethylene diisocyanate or on mixtures of polyurethanes with poly(L-lactide) were used for the preparation of small-caliber vascular grafts [*32*], artificial skin [*33*], and oesophageal prostheses [*34*], and proprietary biodegradable polyurethane elastomers, for designing vascular grafts [*35-37*], pericardial patches [*38*] and porous membranes for the treatment of periodontitis or segmental bone defects [*39,40*]. Biodegradable vascular prostheses induced in animals the growth of functional "neo-arteries" having a cellular structure and compliance similar to those of the natural vessels [*32,35-37*]. The interest in biodegradable polyurethanes received a new momentum in the late nineties [*7-14,19-24*].

The type of monomers used in the syntheses of biodegradable polyurethanes will to a great extent be dependent on the intended application of the material. Hydrophilic polyurethane elastomers are preferred for the preparation of implants to be used in contact with blood [*1*] or as adhesion barriers, although the ratio between the hydrophilic and hydrophobic components in polyurethanes seems to play an important role in the contact of the material surface with blood proteins and cells. The polyurethanes bsed on polyethylene oxide are highly hydrophilic materials. At higher polyethylene oxide content, these polymers in the aqueous environment behave like hydrogels, taking up to 200% of water depending on their chemical composition. They are nonadhesive to proteins, cells and tissues. Thus, polyurethanes with higher amounts of hydrophobic component may be required for scaffolds to be used as porous cancellous bone graft substitutes and for cell culture. It should be kept in mind, however, that hydrophobicity is only one of many characteristics which determine the interaction of polyurethane scaffolds with osteogenic cells and in consequence, its performance as bone substitute [*41*].

The purpose of the present study was to synthesize and characterize linear biodegradable polyurethanes with varying hydrophilic-to-hydrophobic ratios for use as adhesion barriers and porous scaffolds for tissue-engineered implants.

Experimental

Polymer Syntheses

The segmented polyester-ether urethanes with hydrophilic-to-hydrophobic ratios of 30:70, 40:60, 50:50 and 70:30% were synthesized in bulk at 50 to 100°C according to the scheme:

2 O=C=N-R-N=C=O + HO-(R')$_n$-OH → O=C=N-R-NH-CO-O-(R')$_n$-O-OC-HN-R-N=C=O

Diisocyanate Polyol Prepolymer (macrodiisocyanate)

O=C=N-R-NH-CO-O-(R')$_n$-O-OC-HN-R-N=C=O + HO-R"-OH →

Prepolymer Diol

-[-O-R"-O-OC-HN-R-NH-CO-O-(R')$_n$-O-OC-HN-R-NH-CO-O-R"-O-]$_x$-

Polyurethane

The composition and length of segments were varied by using polyols with different molecular weights. The polyols used were poly(ε-caprolactone) (PCL) with molecular weights (MW) 530, 1250, 2000 (Tone™ Polyols, Union Carbide, Danbury, USA, or Aldrich, Milwaukee, USA), poly(ethylene oxide) (PEO) MW=600 and 2000 (Fluka, Buchs, Switzerland), poly(ethylene-propylene-ethylene oxide) Pluronic F-68 MW=8000 (Sigma Chemical, St. Louis, USA), and polyethylene adipate (PEA) MW=1000 (Aldrich). The chain extenders were 1,4-butane diol (1,4-BD), 3-hexyne-2,5-diol (3-HD) and 2-amino-1-butanol (2-AB) (Fluka). The diisocyanates were hexamethylene diisocyanate (HMDI) (Sigma) and isophorone diiscocyanate (IPD) (Fluka). The catalyst used were stannous octoate (Sigma) and dibutyltin dilaurate (Fluka). The polymers were dissolved in dimethylformamide (DMF, Fluka) to obtain a 15 wt-% solution, filtered through S-2 sintered glass filters and cast on glass trays. After solvent evaporation the resulting materials were washed with deionized water, ethanol, dried to constant weight at 50°C under vacuum, dissolved in chloroform, filtered, and cast on glass trays to obtain films with thicknesses in the range of 0.08 to 0.35 mm. The films were stored in desiccators prior to use. Porous scaffolds were prepared by a phase-reverse process from polymer solutions in solvent-nonsolvent systems.

Material Characterization

Viscosity Measurements

Intrinsic viscosities of polymer solutions in DMF were measured at 30°C±0.01° using the Ubbelohde I capillary viscometer. The following constants were used in the Mark-Houwink equation for calculation of molecular weight: $K = 6.80 \times 10^{-5}$ dL/g and $\alpha = 0.86$ [*43*].

Size Exclusion Chromatography (SEC)

Molecular weight distribution and relative molecular weights were determined by SEC analyses carried out on a Waters modular GPC system, consisting of a 510 pump, an U6K injector and the 410 refractive index detector. Data analysis was conducted using the Waters Maxima 820 software package. Correction factors for peak spreading were measured and applied to all molecular weight determinations. A set of three Waters Styragel columns: linear, 10^5 and 10^4 nm maintained at 60°C was used. Calibration was carried out with polystyrene molecular weight standards supplied by Tosoh (Tosoh Corporation, Tokoi, Japan). Polymer samples were kept in a desicator until studied,then dissolved (0.2% w/v), with occasional, gentle swirling every 30 minutes, at 65°C for 90 minutes in solution of lithium chloride in dimethylformamide (0.05 mol/L) followed by filtration through a 0.45 μm Millex SR filter prior to injection (300 μL). Aproximately 120 mg of sample were used to ensure good representation of the polymer. A flow rate of 1.0 mL/min was applied. Three replicate analyses were performed on each polymer sample and the molecular weight values averaged.

Mechanical Properties

An Instron (High Wycombe, Bucks, England) model 4302 tester equipped with a 1 kN load cell operating at a cross-head speed of 200 mm/min and standard Instron pneumatic-action grips cat. no. 2712-003-004 were used to measure the tensile strengths (TS), Young's moduli (E) and elongation at break (ε) of the films. The sample length between the grips was 20 mm. All the values given are means of six measurements (± standard deviation).

Thermal Analysis

A Perkin-Elmer (Norwalk, CONN) differential scanning calorimeter (Pyris DSC-1) calibrated with indium was used for evaluation of the samples' heat transitions. Circular samples with an average weight of 3 to 12 mg were used for the measurements. The samples were scanned at the heating rate of 10°C/min under dry, oxygen free nitrogen flowing at the rate of 50 to 60 ml/min. The samples were scanned from -150 to 200°C.

Scanning Electron Microscopy

A Hitachi (Tokyo, Japan) model S-4100 field emission scanning electron microscope was used to observe the samples sputtered with a 15 nm thick gold-palladium layer. The instrument was operated at 2.0 kV.

Infrared Spectroscopy

Infrared spectra of the polyurethanes were recorded in transmission and reflection modes using a Fourier-Transform Perkin Elmer 2000 FT-IR spectrometer (Beaconsfield, Buckinghamshire, England). An attenuated total reflection (ATR) unit was fitted with KRS-5 crystal (45° entrance angle). The average film thickness was 0.08 mm for transmission and 0.3 mm for reflection measurements, respectively. Thirty scans were taken for each sample.

NMR Analysis

^{1}H-NMR spectra of the polyurethanes in dimethyl sulfoxide (Fluka) were recorded at 27°C using the Bruker 250 MHz nuclear magnetic resonance spectrometer (Bruker, Rheinstetten, Germany). Tetramethylsilane was used as a reference.

Protein Adsorption

Sheep whole blood and bovine albumin solution in phosphate buffer (2 mg/ml, Sigma) was used in the experiments. Polyurethane films 47 x 12 x 0.3 mm were placed in blood or in the albumin solution maintained at 37°C upon stirring. Next, the films coated with the proteins were rinsed three times with distilled water, dried in a vacuum oven at 30°C, fixed on the KRS-5 crystal of the IR-ATR unit, and the IR spectra were recorded. The spectrum of the nontreated film was used as a background. Thirty scans were taken per sample. The amide I region at 1630-1660 cm^{-1} was monitored to assess the proteins adsorbed to the film surface.

Results

Material Characterization

The characteristics of the polyurethanes are listed in Tables 1 and 2, and the typical SEC chromatograms are shown in Fig. 1.

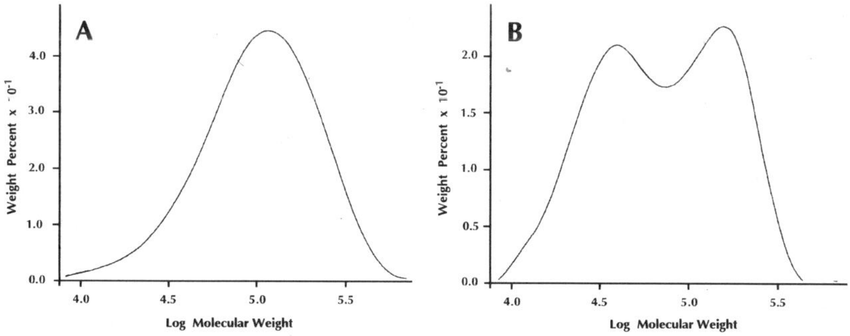

Figure 1 - *SEC chromatograms of polyester-ether urethane elastomers. A, HMDI:PCL 530:PEO 2000:1,4-BD; B, HMDI:PCL 2000:PEO 600:2-AB.*

The molecular weights of the materials listed in Table 1 were estimated from the SEC and the intrinsic viscosity measurements. Two equations were proposed for the calculation of molecular weight from the viscosity measurements in dimethylformamide at 25°C [*42*] and at 30°C [*43*]. Calculation of molecular weights from the equation given in [*42*] yielded values almost five times higher than the values obtained from the SEC data. The values of molecular weights calculated from the equation given in [*43*] were comparable to those obtained from size exclusion chromatography. Hence, the values calculated according to the latter equation were listed in Table 1.

Table 1. *Composition and Molecular Characteristics of Polyurethanes.*

No.	Polyurethane	Content (%)	[η] (dL/g)	M_v	M_w	M_n	M_w/M_n
1	PCL530	100	0.79	53.740	62.480	23.550	2.7
2	PCL1250	100	0.49	31.240	35.800	21.160	1.7
3	PCL2000	100	1.09	78.180	116.900	64.000	1.8
4	PCL530-PEO2000	70:30	0.40	24.420	35.420	20.120	1.8
5	PCL530-PEO2000	50:50	1.70	130.260	142.030	79.140	1.8
6	PCL2000-PEO600	30:70	0.49	31.090	27.930	18.720	1.5
7	PCL2000-PEO600	50:50	1.14	82.340	159.540	91.110	1.8
8	PCL2000-PEO600	70:30	1.18	85.610	92.2100	49.710	1.9
9	PCL2000-PEO600	60:40	1.19	85.860	117.330	42.730	2.7
10	PCL2000-Pluronic F68	70:30	1.34	99.110	129.820	64.400	2.0
11	PEA1000	100	0.71	47.490	-	-	-
12	PCL2000	100	0.41	24.920	-	-	-

Table 2. *Thermal and Mechanical Properties of Polyurethanes.*

No.	Polyurethane	Content (%)	T_{g1} (°C)	T_{g2} (°C)	T_m (°C)	ΔH_m (J/g)	TS (MPa)	E (MPa)	ε (%)
1	PCL530	100	-101.5	-42.5	-	-	40.8	58.8	680
2	PCL1250	100	-106.7	-52.7	28.4	9.3	20.2	20.0	866
3	PCL2000	100	-112.0	-57.6	43.0	23.0	47.2	9.8	723
4	PCL530-PEO2000	70:30	-115.7	-51.4	27.0	33.0	4.0	12.5	121
5	PCL530-PEO2000	50:50	-	-49.0	33.1	54.7	48.6	31.0	842
6	PCL2000-PEO600	30:70	-	-53.8	39.7	12.1	11.0	16.2	706
7	PCL2000-PEO600	50:50	-	-52.6	37.0	25.8	36.6	7.3	795
8	PCL2000-PEO600	70:30	-	-53.3	41.2	17.0	45.0	13.7	736
9	PCL2000-PEO600	60:40	-114.5	-54.8	40.8	41.3	36.4	12.9	723
10	PCL2000-Pluronic F68	70:30	-113.1	-59.6	37.4	46.1	34.5	22.0	957
11	PEA1000	100	-	-40.9	-	-	60.7	72.0	382
12	PCL2000	100	-	-45.8	40.2	36.7	6.4	52.0	100

Polymers were synthesized using: 1 to 8, hexamethylene diiscocyanate and a 1,4-butane diol chain extender; 9 and 10, hexamethylene diisocyanate and 2-amino-1-butanol; 11, isophorone diisocyanate and 3-hexyne-2,5-diol, and 12, isophorone diisocyanate and 1,4-butane diol.

Polyurethane Scaffolds

Scanning electron micrographs of polyurethane membranes are shown in Figs 2A (cross-section) and 2B (surface).

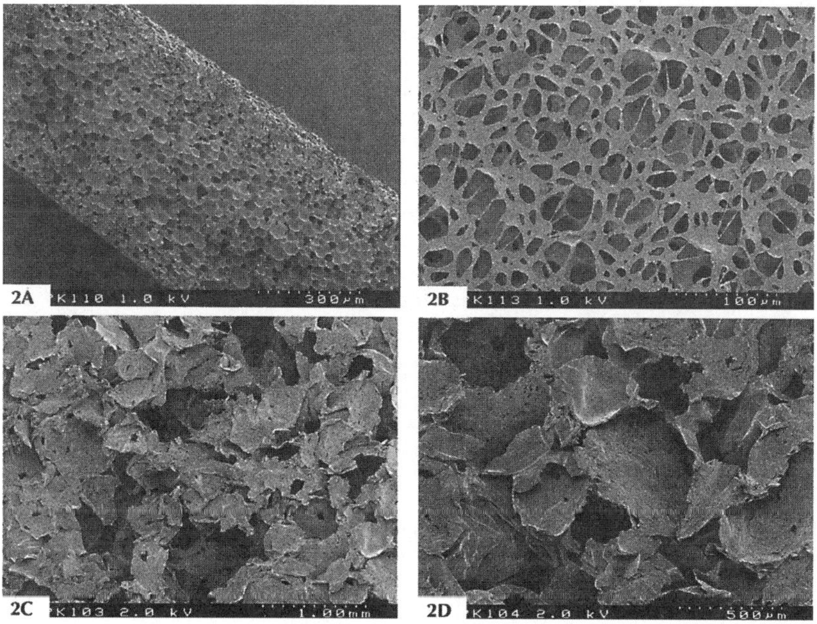

Figure 2 - *Scaffolds from poly(ε-caprolactone urethane). Membrane, 2A, cross-section, 2B, surface; 2C, sponge, 2D, higher magnification of the sample shown in 2C exhibiting small pores in the walls separating the large pores.*

The membrane cross-section exhibits primarily a closed-cell structure while the surface layer consists of the large, interconnected pores with an average pore size in the range of 50 to 100 µm. Sponges shown in Figs 2C and 2D have interconnected pores with an average pore size in the range of 200 to 500 µm. The porosity of the sponges defined, as the ratio of aggregated pore space to the volume of entire mass was 94.6±0.3%. The walls separating the pores are microporous pores ranging from 5 to 50 µm. Liquids, e.g. whole blood easily penetrated the sponges.

Infrared spectroscopy

Typical infrared spectra of selected polyurethanes with various ratios of the ester-to-ether component are shown in Figs 3 to 6. There are distinctive absorption bands at 3363-3322, 2942-2936, 2867-2865, 1732-1720, 1539-1529, 1464, 1365-1349, 1260-1256, 1244-1240, 1171, 1110-1107, 1045, 962, 733 cm^{-1}. The absorption at 3322-3363 cm^{-1} corresponds to hydrogen-bonded -NH groups and a small shoulder at 3445 cm^{-1} can be attributed to nonbonded -NH groups [*44-48*]. The absorption bands at 2936-2942 cm^{-1}

and 2865-2867 cm^{-1} are associated with asymmetric and symmetric $-CH_2$ groups. The strong band at 1732 cm^{-1} in poly(ester urethane) is assigned to the -C=O groups. In poly(ester-ether urethanes) the increase of polyether diol chain length (molecular weight) and the decrease of polyester molecular weight resulted in a shift of the bonded -NH peak at 3328 cm^{-1} and the ester carbonyl peak at 1732 cm^{-1} in the direction of lower frequencies and the appearance of the -C=O band at 1685 cm^{-1}. The appearance of this band and a shift of the -NH band towards lower frequencies indicate an improvement in the hydrogen bonding network between -NH, -C=O and ether -O- groups [*45*]. The amide II absorption appears at 1531 cm^{-1} for poly(ester urethane) and at 1540 cm^{-1} for poly(ester-ether urethanes), respectively. The various modes of $-CH_2$ vibrations are manifested by the bands at 1464, 1419, 1396, 1365, 1350, 1295 1540 cm^{-1}. The amide III aliphatic R-NH-COO- groups are manifested by the bands at 1260-1256 cm^{-1} [*45*]. In poly(ester-ether urethanes) synthesized in the present study this band appeared only in the materials having the ether polyol component with a molecular weight of 2000.

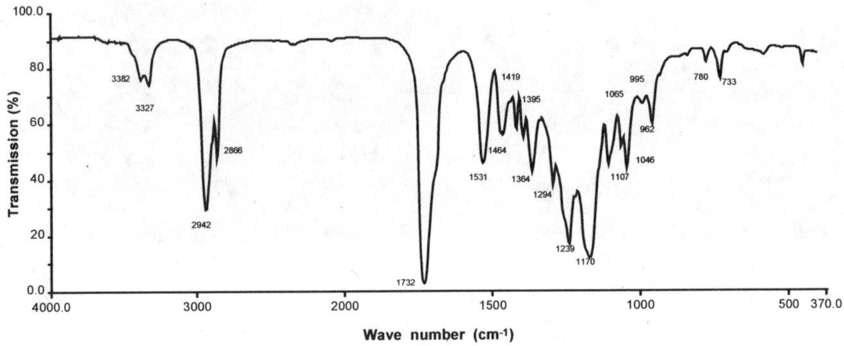

Figure 3 - *Infrared spectrum of a polyester urethane elastomer HMDI:PCL 2000:1,4-BD.*

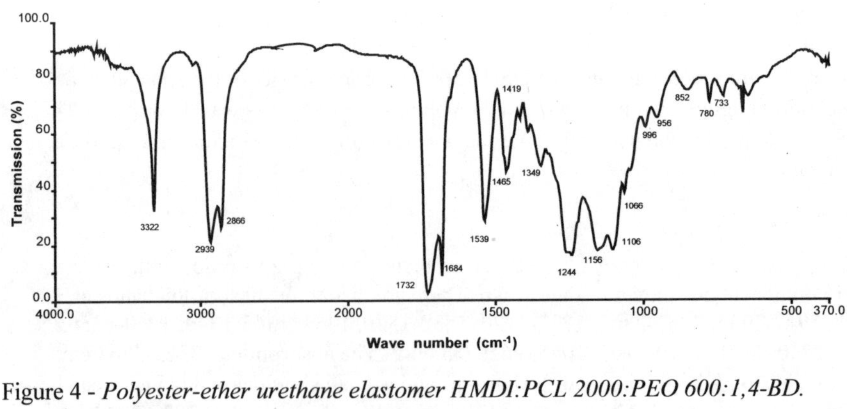

Figure 4 - *Polyester-ether urethane elastomer HMDI:PCL 2000:PEO 600:1,4-BD.*

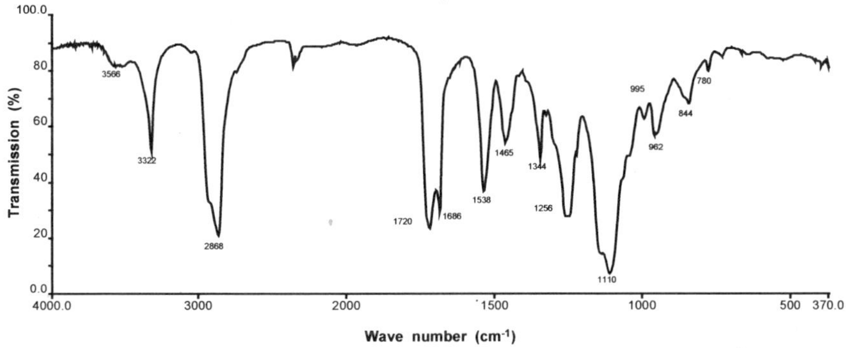

Figure 5 - *Polyester-ether urethane elastomer HMDI:PCL 530:PEO 2000:1,4-BD.*

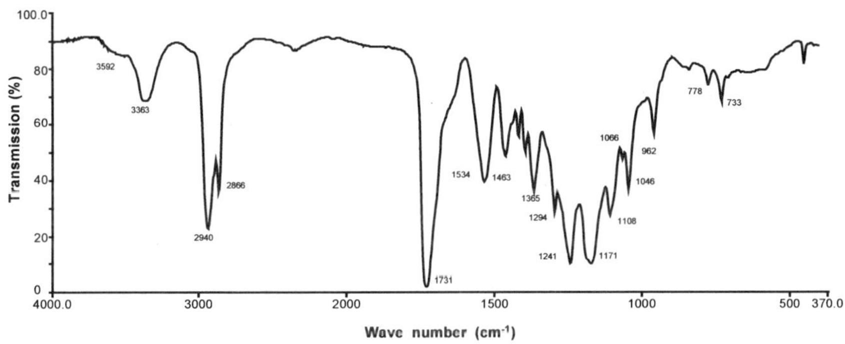

Figure 6 - *Polyester-ether urethane elastomer HMDI:PCL 2000:PEO 600:2-AB.*

The bands at 1244-1240, 1172-1170, 1066-1063 and 760-630 cm^{-1} were only present in the materials synthesized from polycaprolactone diols and/or from the mixtures of polycaprolactone and polyethylene oxide diols with lower molecular weights up to 600.These bands are assigned to the stretching vibration of the ester group -CO-O-C- in poly(ester urethanes) [*47*]. The band at 1110-1106 cm^{-1} is attributed to the =C-O stretching for poly(ester urethanes) (weak), and to the stretching of the ether -C-O-C- group for poly(ester-ether urethanes) (very strong). The intensity of this band increases with the increasing content and length of the polyether component in the polymer.

NMR

The representative ^{1}H-NMR spectrum of poly(ε-caprolactone-ethylene oxide urethane) is shown in Fig. 7. The polymer was obtained using polycaprolactone- and polyethylene diols with a molecular weight of 530 and 2000, respectively. The polyols were mixed together at 1:1 ratio. There are seven characteristic peaks in the spectrum, at 1.2 - 1.6

(-C$\underline{H}_2$-), 2.25-2.30(-C$\underline{H}_2$-CO-O-), 2.92-2.94(-C$\underline{H}_2$-NH-CO-), 3.61(-C$\underline{H}_2$-O-), 3.9-4.2 (-C$\underline{H}_2$-O-CO-), 4.5(-CH_2-OH), and 7.0(-N$\underline{H}$-CO-) ppm. As it might be expected the intensity of peaks at 2.25-2.30 ppm was highest for poly(ester urethanes) obtained from poly(ε-caprolactone) diol with a highest molecular weight (2000), and lowest for poly(ester-ether urethanes) with a highest molecular weight (2000) and highest content of poly(ethylene oxide) (50%). This indicates that the synthesized materials had the intended hydrophilic-to-hydrophobic ratio.

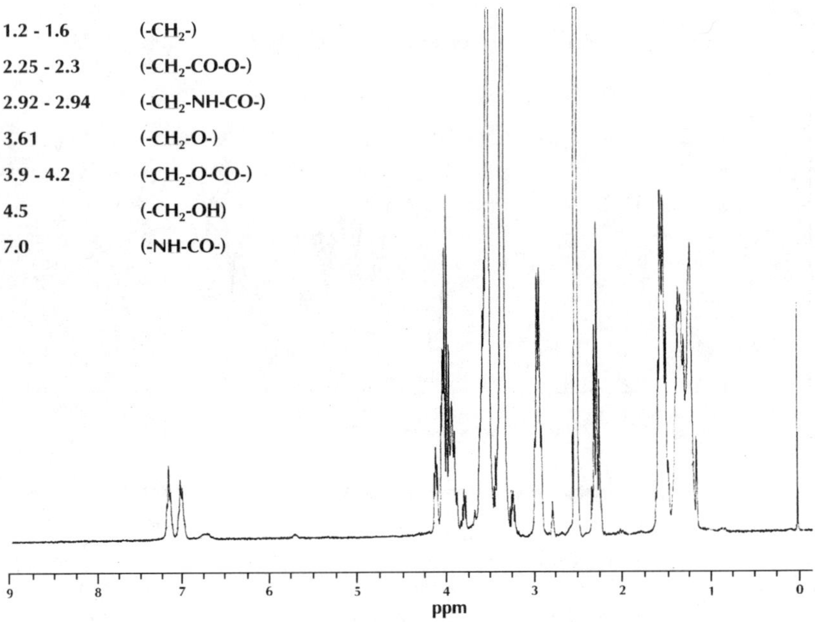

Figure 7 - *¹H-NMR spectrum of polyester-ether urethane elastomer HMDI:PCL 530: PEO 2000:1,4-BD.*

Protein adsorption

Exemplary infrared spectra of selected polyurethanes exposed to whole blood are shown in Fig. 8 A and B. A broad shoulder at 1640 cm^{-1} (amide I region) which developed in poly(ester urethanes) exposed to blood is an indication of protein adsorption to the material [*49-55*]. There was no protein adsorption to the poly(ester-ether urethanes) during the experiment.

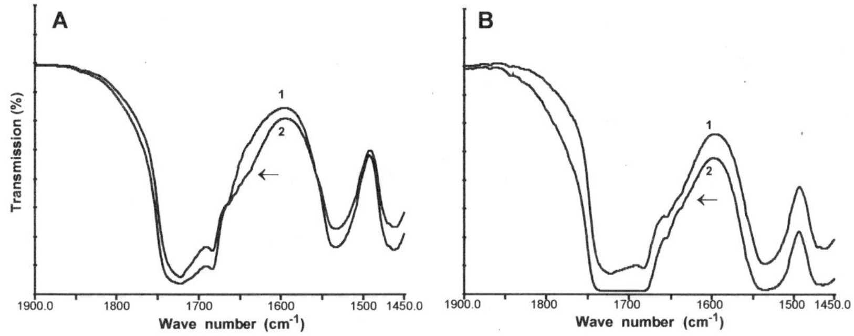

Figure 8 - *FTIR spectra of A, poly(ester urethane); and B, poly(ester-ether urethane) 30/70% exposed to whole blood for 0 hours (1) and 18 hours (2), respectively.*

Discussion

Interest in biodegradable polymers for medical applications is steadily increasing. Typical applications are in sutures, drug delivery devices, internal fixation of bone fractures and scaffolds for tissue engineering, just to mention a few. The suitability of a given degradable polymer for a particular implantable device depends on the properties associated with its chemical composition, molecular weight, processability, degradation rate, not to mention the mechanical properties to be developed in the implant.

Rigid polymers such as polyhydroxyacids are used for internal fixation of bone fractures, porous membranes for the treatment of bone defects, matrices for cells and cancellous bone substitutes [*56-59*]. Segmented degradable polyurethanes can find applications in a number of implants if the implant elasticity and/or controlled hydrophobic-to-hydrophilic ratio are required [*1,2*]. Hydrophilic materials nonadherent to proteins, cells and tissues could be used for adhesion barriers. More hydrophobic materials which attract proteins and support the attachment and growth of particular cells can potentially be used in tissue and organ regeneration scaffolds.

Biodegradable polyurethanes with varying hydrophilicity can be obtained from mixtures of poly(ε-caprolactone) and poly(ethylene oxide) diols and various chain extenders. Poly(ε-caprolactone) is a biocompatible, slowly degrading polymer [*60*]. Its degradation can be facilitated by incorporating labile units such as polyethylene oxide, glycolide or lactides in the polymer chain [*61-66*]. Poly(ethylene oxide) and (ethylene oxide-propylene oxide-ethylene oxide) triblock copolymers have properties of resisting protein and cell adhesion [*55,67-74*]. Polyurethanes based on poly(ε-caprolactone) diols are hydrophobic, strong and hydrolyze at low rates [*75,76*], while polyurethanes from poly(ethylene oxide) diols are hydrophilic [*67,77*], susceptible to hydrolysis [*31,78*] and have mechanical properties inferior to those of polycaprolactone materials.

The use in the present study of mixtures of poly(ε-caprolactone) and poly(ethylene oxide) diols instead of the individual polyols [*31*] allowed for the preparation of polyurethanes with controllable degradation rates [*78*] and varying hydrophobic-to-hydrophilic ratios. The successful incorporation of the ether unit in the polymer molecule was assessed from the NMR measurements. The intensity of ^{1}H-NMR peaks at 2.25-2.30 (-C$\underline{H}_2$-CO-O-) and 3.9-4.2 ppm (-C$\underline{H}_2$-O-CO-) was highest for the poly(ε-caprolactone urethane) obtained from the PCL diol with a highest MW=2000. The peak intensity decreased with an increasing amount and a molecular weight of the PEO diol in the polyols mixture used in the synthesis, reaching the lowest value for the poly(ε-caprolactone-ethylene oxide urethane) obtained from the PCL and PEO diols with molecular weights of 530 and 2000, respectively, mixed at the ratio of 1:1. The increase in the PEO molecular weight, and the decrease in the PCL molecular weight in the polyols mixture resulted in a shift of the bonded -NH peak at 3328 cm^{-1} and the ester carbonyl peak at 1732 cm^{-1} in the direction of lower frequencies, and the appearance of the -C=O band at 1685 cm^{-1}. This is indicative of the improvement of hydrogen bonding between the -NH, -C=O and ether -O- groups [*45*]. The improvement in hydrogen bonding was not accompanied by an evident enhancement of the materials mechanical properties [*1*], the latter being comparable to those of commercial and experimental polyurethanes [*1,31,79*]. The materials in the study synthesized from polyols with a lower molecular weight had higher tensile strengths and moduli, but lower elongation at break than the corresponding materials synthesized from polyols with higher molecular weights. A similar trend was also reported for segmented polyurethanes based on polycaprolactone diols and aromatic and/or cycloaliphatic diisocyanates [*79*]. The molecular weights of the polyurethanes obtained in the study were similar to the values given in the literature for segmented polyurethanes produced using aliphatic and/or aromatic diisocyanates and various polyester or polyether diols [*1,80*]. All the materials synthesized using 1,4-butane diol or 2-amino-1-butanol showed an unimodal molecular weight distribution except for the polyurethane from HMDI, PCL 2000, PEO 600 and (2-AB) chain extender which exhibited a bimodal distribution. The reasons are not clear although it might be speculated that at the given length of the ether and ester segments the presence of the amino group on the chain extender may enhance phase segregation. Almost all the samples showed thermal transitions at about -110°C and -50°C which can be assigned to local motions of -$(CH_2)_4$- units and the glass transition of the soft segments, respectively [*81*]. Poly(ester-ether urethanes) showed melting endotherms at about 40°C for the materials obtained from PCL 2000 and PEO 600, and about 30°C for the materials from PCL 530 and PEO 2000. These endotherms correspond to the melting and reorganization of the soft segment domains, which processes have no assessable consequences for structural properties of devices at body temperature. Poly(ε-caprolactone urethane) from PCL 530 or from poly(ethylene adipate) 1000 did not exhibit melting endotherms on the DSC thermograms. This may be due to the low molecular weight of the polyol and a high hard segment content [*79*].

The poly(ester urethanes) obtained in the study adsorbed blood proteins while poly(ester-ether urethanes) did not. This property of poly(ester-ether urethanes) was independent of the ether molecular weight and its content in the polyols mixture. The use of ether-ester polyol mixture in the synthesis of biodegradable polyurethanes can be another route to produce surfaces with required hydrophilic-to-hydrophobic ratios preventing unwanted adhesion of proteins, cells and tissues. The chemical incorporation of PEO or PEO-PPO-PEO surfactants with prevailing PEO content into the polymer chain may allow for more predictable control of the surface adhesive properties than the simple surface coating with these easily washable components.

Poly(ester urethanes) and poly(ester-ether urethanes) dissolved in good solvents such as tetrahydrofuran or dimethylene sulfoxide containing hydrogen-bonding nonsolvents were easily processed into porous scaffolds such as membranes and sponges using salt-leaching and/or phase-inverse techniques. Preliminary tests showed that osteoblasts attach to porous scaffolds from poly(ester urethanes) suggesting that the scaffold could potentially be used as cancellous bone substitute. Elastomeric porous bone substitute which expands in the defect may ensure a better contact with bone promoting the migration of osteogenic cells and new bone formation.

Acknowledgment

The help of Prof. Stefan Polowinski, D.Sc.,Ph.D., of Department of Physical Chemistry of Polymers, Technical University of Lodz, Poland in interpretation of NMR data is gratefully acknowledged.

References

[1] Lelach, M. D., and Cooper, S. L., "*Polyurethanes in Medicine*," CRC Press, Boca Raton, FL, 1986.

[2] Gogolewski, S., "Selected Topics in Biomedical Polyurethanes. A review," *Colloid & Polymer Science,* Vol. 267, 1989, pp. 757-785.

[3] Gogolewski, S., "Biomedical Polyurethanes," in *"Desk Reference of Functional Polymers. Syntheses and Applications,"* R. Arshady, Ed., American Chemical Society, Washington, DC, 1996, pp. 657-698.

[4] Gogolewski, S., "*In vitro* and *in vivo* Molecular Stability of Medical Polyurethanes: A Review," in "*Trends in Polymer Sciences,"* J. Menon, Ed., Trivandrum, India, Vol. 1, 1991, pp. 47-61.

[5] Anderson, J. M., Hiltner, A., Wiggins, M. J., Schubert, M. A., Collier, T. O., Kao, W. J., and Mathur, A. B., "Recent Advances in Biomedical Polyurethane Biostability and Biodegradation," *Polymer International*, Vol. 46, 1998, pp. 163-171.

[6] Gogolewski, S., and Pennings, A. J., "Biodegradable Materials of Polylactides. IV. Porous Biomedical Materials Based on Mixtures of Polylactides and Polyurethanes," *Makromolekulare Chemie, Rapid Communications,* Vol. 3, 1982, pp. 839-845.

[7] Hiljanen-Vainio, M., Kylmä, J., Hiltunen, K., and Seppälä, J. V., "Impact Modification of Lactic Acid Based Poly(ester-urethanes) by Blending," *Journal of Applied Polymer Science,* Vol. 63, 1997, pp. 1335-1343.

[8] Kylmä, J., Härkönen, M., and Seppälä, J. V., "The Modification of Lactic Acid Based Poly(ester-urethane) by Copolymerization," *Journal of Applied Polymer Science,* Vol. 63, 1997, 1865-1872.

[9] Hiltunen, K., Seppälä , J. V., and Härkönen, M., "Lactic Acid Based Poly(ester-urethane)s: The Effects of Different Polymerization Conditions on the Polymer Structure and Properties," *Journal of Applied Polymer Science,* Vol. 64, 1997, pp. 865-873.

[10] Hiljanen-Vainio, M., Heino, M., and Seppälä, J. V., "Reinforcement of Biodegradable Poly(ester-urethane) with Fillers," *Polymer*, Vol. 39, 1998, pp. 865-872.

[11] Hiltunen, K., Tuominen, J, and Seppälä, J. V., "Hydrolysis of Lactic Acid Based Poly(ester-urethane)s," *Polymer International,* Vol. 47, 1998, pp. 186-192.

[12] Saad, B., Hirt, T. D., Welti, M., Uhlschmid, G. K., Neuenschwander, P., and Suter, U. W., "Development of Degradable Polyesterurethanes for Medical Applications: *In vitro* and *In vivo* Evaluations," *Journal of Biomedical Materials Research,* Vol. 36, 1997, pp. 65-74.

[13] Ciardelli, G., Saad, B., Lendlein, A., Neuenschwander, P., and Suter, U. W., "Synthesis of Fluorescence-Labelled Short-Chain Polyester Segments for the Investigation of Bioresorbable Poly(ester-urethane)," *Macromolecular Chemistry and Physics*, Vol. 198, 1997, pp. 1481-1498.

[14] Saad, B., Ciardelli, G., Matter, S., Welti, M., Uhlschmid, G. K., Neuenschwander, P., and Suter, U. W., "Degradable and Highly Porous Polyesterurethane Foam as Biomaterial: Effects and Phagocytosis of Degradation Products in Osteoblasts," *Journal of Biomedical Materials Research,* Vol. 39, 1998, pp. 594-602.

[15] Lipatova, T. E., Pkhakadze, G. A., Vsilchenko, D. V., Vorona, V. V., and Shilov, V. V., "Structural Peculiarities of Block Copolyurethanes with Peptide Links as Rigid Block Extenders," *Biomaterials*, Vol. 4, 1983, pp. 201-204.

[16] Sosa, K., Mori, A., Sisiodo, M., and Imanishi, Y., "Synthesis of Polyurethanes Containing L-serine Dipeptide and their Use as Materials for Biomedical Films," *Biomaterials,* Vol. 6, 1985, 312-324.

[17] Mori, A., Imanishi, Y., Ito, T., and Sakaoku, K., "Effect of Thermal Treatment on the Structure and the Biomedical Properties of Polyurethane Film Containing Dipeptides of L-serine," *Biomaterials*, Vol. 6, 1985, 325-337.

[18] Lipatova, T. E., Pkhakadze, G. A., Snegirev, A. I., Vorona, V. V., and Shilov, V. V., "Supermolecular Organization of Some Polyurethanes Containing Sugar Derivatives in the Main Chain," *Journal of Biomedical Materials Research,* Vol. 18, 1984, pp. 129-136.

[19] Hashimoto, K., Wilbullucksanakul, S., and Okada, M., "Polyaddition of Saccharic Dilactones with Hexamethylene Diisocyanate," *Makromolekulare Chemie, Rapid Communication*, Vol. 14, 1993, 591-595.

[20] Hashimoto, K., Wilbullucksanakul, S., and Okada, M., "Macromolecular Synthesis from Saccharic Lactones. Polyaddition of D-Glucaro- and D-Manaro-1,4:6,3-dilactones with Diisocyanates and Hydrolyzability of the Resulting Polyurethanes Having Dilactone Rings in the Main Chains," *Journal of Polymer Science, A: Polymer Chemistry*, Vol. 33, 1995, pp. 1495-1503.

[21] Wilbullucksanakul, S., Hashimoto, K., and Okada, M., "Synthesis of Polyurethanes from Saccharide-Derived Diols and Diisocyanates and their Hydrolyzability," *Macromolecular Chemistry and Physics*, Vol. 197, 1996, 135-146.

[22] Wilbullucksanakul, S., Hashimoto, K., and Okada, M., "Swelling Behavior and Controlled Release of New Hydrolyzable Poly(ether urethane) Gels Derived from Saccharide and L-lysine Derivatives and Poly(ethylene glycol)," *Macromolecular Chemistry and Physics*, Vol. 197, 1996, 1865-1876.

[23] Wilbullucksanakul, S., Hashimoto, K., and Okada, M., "Hydrolysis and Release Behavior of Hydrolyzable Poly(ether urethane) Gels Derived from Saccharide-, L-lysine Derivatives, and Poly(propylene glycol)," *Macromolecular Chemistry and Physics*, Vol. 198, 1997, 305-319.

[24] Sreenivasan, K., "On the Biostability of a Novel β-cyclodextrin Based Hydrophilic Polyurethane," *Polymer Degradation and Stability*, Vol. 53, 1996, pp. 73-77.

[25] Bruin, P., Veenstra, G. J., Nijenhuis, A. J., and Pennings, A. J., "Design and Synthesis of Biodegradable Poly(ester-urethane) Elastomer Networks Composed of Non-Toxic Building Blocks," *Makromolekulare Chemie, Rapid Communication,* Vol. 9, 1988, pp. 589-594.

[26] Pitt, C. G., Gu, Z. W., Ingram, P., and Hendren, R. W., "The Synthesis of Biodegradable Polymers with Functional Side Chains," *Journal of Polymer Science, A, Polymer Chemistry*, Vol. 25, 1987, pp. 955-966.

[27] Storey, R. F., Herring, K. R., and Hoffman, D. C., "Hydroxy-Terminated Poly(ε-Caprolactone-co-δ-Valerolactone) Oligomers: Synthesis, Characterization, and Polyurethane Network Formation," *Journal of Polymer Science, A: Polymer Chemistry*, Vol. 29, 1991, 1759-1777.

[28] Shi, F. Y., Wang, L. F., Tashev, E., and Leong, K. W., "Syntesis and Characterization of Hydrolytically Labile Poly(phosphoester-urethanes)," in "*Polymeric Drugs and Drug Delivery Systems*," R. L. Dunn and R. M. Ottenbrite, Eds. *ACS Symposium Series,* Vol. 469, 1991, pp. 141-154, American Chemical Society, Washington, DC.

[29] Storey, R. F., Wiggins, J. S., and Mauritz, K. A., "Bioabsorbable Composites. II. Nontoxic, L-lysine-Based Poly(ester-urethane) Matrix Composites," *Polymer Composites*, Vol. 14, 1993, pp. 17-25.

[30] Storey, R. F., Wiggins, J. S., and Puckett, A. D., "Hydrolyzable Poly(ester-urethane) Networks from L-Lysine Diisocyanate and D,L-Lactide/ε-Caprolactone Homo- and Copolyester Triols," *Journal of Polymer Science, A: Polymer Chemistry*, Vol. 32, 1994, pp. 2345-2363.

[31] Skarja, G. A., and Woodhouse, K. A., "Synthesis and Characterization of Degradable Polyurethane Elastomers Containing an Amino Acid-Based Chain Extender," *Journal of Biomaterials Science, Polymer Edition*, Vol. 9, 1998, pp. 271-295.

[32] Gogolewski, S., Pennings, A. J., Lommen, E., Nieuwenhuis, P., and Wildevuur, Ch. R. H., "Growth of a Neo-artery Induced by a Biodegradable Polymeric Vascular Prosthesis," *Makromolekulare Chemie, Rapid Communication,* Vol. 4, 1983, pp. 213-219.

[33] Gogolewski, S., and Pennings, A. J., "An Artificial Skin Based on Biodegradable Mixtures of Polylactides and Polyurethanes for Full-thickness Wound Covering," *Makromolekulare Chemie, Rapid Communication,* Vol. 4, 1983, pp. 675-680.

[34] Wang, F., Nieuwenhuis, P., Gogolewski, S., Pennings, A. J., and Wildevuur, R. Ch. H., "Oesophageal Prosthesis," in *"Progress in Biomedical Engineering, Polyurethanes in Biomedical Engineering,"* H. Planck, G. Egbers, and I. Syré, Eds., Vol. 1, 1984, pp. 317-332.

[35] Gogolewski, S., and Galletti, G., "Degradable Vascular Prosthesis from Segmented Polyurethanes," *Colloid & Polymer Science,* Vol. 264, 1986, pp. 854-858.

[36] Gogolewski, S., Galletti, G., and Ussia, G., "Polyurethane Vascular Prosthesis in Pigs," *Colloid & Polymer Science,* Vol. 265, 1987, pp. 774-778.

[37] Galletti, G., Gogolewski, S., Ussia, G., and Faruggia, F., "Long-term Patency of Regenerated Neoaortic Wall Following the Implant of a Fully Biodegradable Polyurethane Prosthesis: Experimental Lipid Diet Model in Pigs," *Annals of Vascular Surgery,* Vol. 3, 1989, 236-243.

[38] Gogolewski, S., Walpoth, B., and Rheiner, P., "Polyurethane Microporous Membranes as Pericardial Substitutes," *Colloid & Polymer Science,* Vol. 265, 1987, pp. 971-977.

[39] Warrer, K., Karring, T., Nyman, S., and Gogolewski, S., "Guided Tissue Regeneration Using Biodegradable Membranes of Polylactic Acid or Polyurethane," *Journal of Clinical Periodontology,* Vol. 19, 1992, pp. 633-640.

[40] Farsϕ-Nielsen, F., Karring, T., and Gogolewski, S., "Biodegradable Guide for Bone Regeneration. Polyurethane Membranes Tested in Rabbit Radius Defects," *Acta Orthopeadica Scandinavica,* Vol. 63, 1992, pp. 66-69.

[41] Gogolewski, S., Wieling, R., and Gorna, K., "The treatment of Segmental Diaphyseal Defects in the Sheep Tibiae Using Three-dimensional Porous Scaffolds from Biodegradable Polyurethanes," *in preparation.*

[42] Chang, Y. J. P., and Wilkes, G. L. "Superstructure in Segmented Polyether-Urethanes," *Journal of Polymer Science: Polymer Physics Edition,* Vol. 13, 1975, pp. 455-476.

[43] Seefried, C. G., Jr., Koleske J. V., Critchfield, F. E., and Pfaffenberger, C. R., "Thermoplastic Urethane Elastomers. VI. Dilute Solution Properties in Various Solvents," *Journal of Polymer Science, Polymer Physics Edition*, Vol. 18, 1980, pp. 817-828.

[44] Seymour, R. W., Estes, G. M., and Cooper, S. L. "Infrared Studies of Segmented Polyurethane Elastomers. I. Hydrogen Bonding," *Macromolecules*, Vol. 3, 1970, pp. 579-583.

[45] Hummel, D. O., Ellinghorst, G., Khatachatryan, A., and Stenzenberger, H.-D., "Segmented Copolyethers with Urethane and Urea or Semicarbazide Systems II," *Die Angewandte Makromolekulare Chemie*, Vol. 82, 1979, pp. 129-148.

[46] Wilhelm, C., and Gardette, J.-L., "Infrared Analysis of the Photochemical Behaviour of Segmented Polyurethanes: 1. Aliphatic poly(ester-urethane)," *Polymer*, Vol. 38, 1997, pp. 4019-4031.

[47] Srichatrapimuk, V. W., and Cooper, S. L., "Infrared Thermal Analysis of Polyurethane Block Polymers," *Journal of Macromolecular Science-Physics*, Vol. B15, 1978, pp. 267-311.

[48] Bellamy, L. J., "*The Infra-red Spectra of Complex Molecules,*" Chapman & Hall, London, 1975, pp. 203-220, 231-261.

[49] Matsui, T., Tanaka, S., Akaike, T., Sakurai, Y., Nitadori, Y., Kataoka, K., and Tsuruta, T., "Brief Communication. Study of Plasma Proteins Adsorbed on Polymer Surfaces by Fourier Transform Infrared Spectrometry," *Journal of Bioengineering*, Vol. 2, 1978, pp. 539-541.

[50] Gendreau, R. M., Leininger, R. I., Winter, S., and Jakobsen, R. J., "Fourier Transform Infrared Spectroscopy for Protein-Surface Studies," in "*Advances in Chemistry,*" Series No. 199, 1982, pp. 371-394, S.L. Cooper, Ed., American Chemical Society, Washington, DC.

[51] Gendreau, R. M., "Breaking the One Second Barrier: Fast Kinetics of Protein Adsorption by FT-IR," *Applied Spectroscopy*, Vol. 36, 1982, pp. 47-49.

[52] Sato, H., Morimoto, H., and Nakaima, Y., "Study on Interaction between Plasma Proteins and Polymer Surfaces," *Polymer Journal*, Vol. 16, 1984, pp. 1-8.

[53] Pitt, W. G., and Cooper, S. L., FTIR-ATR Studies of the Effect of Shear Rate upon Albumin Adsorption on Polyurethaneurea," *Biomaterials*, Vol. 7, 1986, pp. 340-347.

[54] Pitt, W. G., Grasel, T. G., and Cooper, S. L., Albumin Adsorption on Alkyl Chain Derivatized Polyurethanes," *Biomaterials*, Vol. 9, 1988, pp. 36-46.

[55] Gombotz, W. R., Guanghui, W., Horbett, T. A., and Hoffman, A. S., "Protein Adsorption to Poly(ethylene oxide) Surfaces," *Journal of Biomedical Materials Research*, Vol. 25, 1991, pp. 1547-1567.

[56] Gogolewski, S., Resorbable Polymers for Internal Fixation," *Clinical Materials*, Vol. 10, 1992, pp. 13-20.

[57] Pineda, L. M., Büsing, M., Meinig, R. P., and Gogolewski, S., "Bone Regeneration with Resorbable Polymeric Membranes. III. Effect of Poly(L-lactide) Membrane Pore Size on the Bone Healing Process in Large Defects," *Journal of Biomedical Materials Research*, Vol. 31, 1996, pp. 385-394.

[58] Gugala, Z., and Gogolewski, S., "Regeneration of Segmental Diaphyseal Defects in Sheep Tibiae Using Resorbable Polymeric Membranes: A Preliminary Study," *Journal of Orthopaedic Trauma*, Vol. 13, 1999, pp. 187-195.

[59] Gogolewski, S., and Wieling, R., "Regeneration of Bone in Large Segmental Diaphyseal Defects Using Bioresorbable Polymeric Scaffolds," *ORS 2000 Annual Meeting,* submitted.

[60] Schindler, A., Jeffcoat, R., Kimmel, G. L., Pitt, C. G., Wall, M. E., and Zweidinger, R., "Biodegradable Polymers for Sustained Drug Delivery, in: "*Contemporary Topics in Polymer Science*", Eds. Pearce, E. M., and Schaefgen, J. R. Plenum Press, New York, Vol. 2, 1977, pp. 251-289.

[61] Bogdanov, B., Vidts, A., van den Bulcke, A., Verbeeck, R., and Schacht, E., "Synthesis and Thermal Properties of Poly(ethylene glycol)-Poly(ε-caprolactone) Copolymers," *Polymer*, Vol. 39, 1998, pp. 1631-1636.

[62] Tjong, S. C., and Bei, J. Z., "Degradation Behavior of Poly(caprolactone)-Poly(ethylene glycol) Block Copolymer/Low-Density Polyethylene Blends," *Polymer Engineering and Science*, Vol. 38, 1998, pp. 392-402.

[63] Pitt, C. G., Gratzl, M. M., Kimmel, G. L., Surles, J., and Schindler, A., Aliphatic Polyesters. II. The Degradation of Poly(DL-lactide), Poly(ε-caprolactone), and their Copolymers *In vivo*," *Biomaterials,* Vol. 2, 1981, pp. 215-220.

[64] Kricheldorf, H. R., Mang, T., and Jonté, J. M., "Polylactones. 1. Copolymerization of Glycolide and ε-Caprolactone," *Macromolecules*, Vol. 17, 1984, pp. 2173-2181.

[65] Sawhney, A. S., and Hubbell, J. A., "Rapidly Degraded Terpolymers of DL-Lactide, Glycolide, and ε-Caprolactone with Increased Hydrophylicity by Copolymerization with Polyethers," *Journal of Biomedical Matererials Research*, Vol. 24, 1990, pp. 1397-1411.

[66] Bezwada, R. S., Jemiolkowski, D. D., Lee, I. Y., Agarwal, V., Persivale, J., Trenka-Benthin, S., Erneta, M., Suryadervara, J., Yang, A., and Liu, S., "Monocryl® Suture, a New Ultra-Pliable Absorbable Monofilament Suture," *Biomaterials*, Vol. 16, 1995, pp. 1141-1148.

[67] Merill, E. W., and Salzman, E. W., "Polyethylene Oxide as Biomaterial," *American Society for Artificial Internal Organs Journal*, Vol. 6, 1983, pp. 60-64.

[68] Amiji, M., and Park, K., "Prevention of Protein Adsorption and Platelet Adhesion on Surfaces by PEO/PPO/PEO Triblock Copolymers," Biomaterials, Vol. 13, 1992, pp. 682-692.

[69] Ng, C. L., Lee, H. K., and Li, S. F. Y, "Prevention of Protein Adsorption on Surfaces by Polyethylene Oxide-Polypropylene Oxide-Polyethylene Oxide Triblock Copolymers in Capillary Electrophoresis," *Journal of Chromatography*, Vol. A 659, 1994, pp. 427-434.

[70] Li, J.T., Carlsson, J., Lin, J. N., and Caldwell, K. D., "Chemical Modification of Surface Active Poly(ethylene oxide)-Poly(propylene oxide) Triblock Copolymers," *Bioconjugate Chemistry*, Vol. 7, 1996, pp. 592-599.

[71] Neff, J. A., Caldwell, K. D., and Tresco, P. A., "A Novel Method for Surface Modification to Promote Cell Attachment to Hydrphobic Substrates," *Journal of Biomedical Materials Research*, Vol. 40, 1998, pp. 511-519.

[72] Dewez, J.-L., Schneider, Y.-J., and Rouxhet, P. G., "Coupled Influence of Substratum Hydrophilicity and Surfactant on Epithelial Cell Adhesion," *Journal of Biomedical Materials Research*, Vol. 30, 1996, pp. 373-383.

[73] Dewez, J.-L., Lhoest, J.-B., Detrait, E., Berger, V., Dupont-Gillain, C. C., Vincent, L.-M., Schneider, Y.-J., Bertrand, P., and Rouxhet, P. G., "Adhesion of Mammalian Cells to Polymer Surfaces: From Physical Chemistry of Surfaces to Selective Adhesion on Defined Patterns," *Biomaterials*, Vol. 19, 1998, pp. 1441-1445.

[74] Green, R. J., Davies, M. C., Roberts, C. J., and Tendler, S. J. B., "A surface Plasmon Resonance Study of Albumin Adsorption to PEO-PPO-PEO Triblock Copolymers," *Journal of Biomedical Materials Research*, Vol. 42, 1998, pp. 165-171.

[75] Schollenberger, C. S., and Stewart, F. D.,"Thermoplastic Polyurethane Hydrolysis Stability," *Journal of Elastoplastics*, Vol. 3, 1971, pp. 28-56.

[76] Tang, Y. W., Santerre, J. P., Labow, R. S., and Taylor, D. G., "Use of Surface-Modifying Macromolecules to Enhance the Biostability of Segmented Polyurethanes," *Journal of Biomedical Materials Research*, Vol. 35, 1997, pp. 371-381.

[77] Gananou, Y., Hild, G., and Rempp, P., " Hydrophilic Polyurethane Networks Based on Poly(ethylene oxide): Synthesis, Characterization, and Properties, Ptential Applications as Biomaterials," *Macromolecules*, Vol. 17, 1984, pp. 945-952.

[78] Gorna, K., and Gogolewski, S., "*In vitro* Degradation and Calcification of Biodegradable Polyurethanes Based on Mixtures of Poly(ε-caprolactone) and Poly(ethylene oxide) Diols and Various Chain Extenders," *submitted.*

[79] Van Bogart, J. W. C., Gibson, P. E., and Cooper, S. L., "Structure-Property Relationships in Polycaprolactone-Polyurethanes," *Journal of Polymer Science: Polymer Edition*, Vol. 21, 1983, pp. 65-95.

[80] Chen, C. T., Eaton, R. F., Chang, Y. J., and Tobolsky, A. V., "Synthesis, Characterization, and Permeation Properties of Polyether-Based Polyurethanes," *Journal of Applied Polymer Science*, Vol. 16, 1972, pp. 2105-2114.

[81] Silver, J. H., Myers, C. W., Lim, F., and Cooper, S. L., "Effect of Polyol Molecular Weight on the Physical Properties and Haemocompatibility of Polyurethanes Containing Polyethylene Oxide Macroglycols," *Biomaterials*, Vol. 15, 1994, pp. 695-704.

[82] Shutov, F. A., "Cellular Structure and Properties of Foamed Polymers," in "*Handbook of Polymeric Foams and Foam Technology*," D. Klempner, and K. C. Frisch, Eds., Hanser Publishers, Munich, 1991, pp. 17-46.

Meng Deng,[1] Jacqueline M. Allan,[1] Joel T. Corbett,[1] and Shalaby W. Shalaby[1]

Effects of Thermal History and Physical Aging on Thermal Properties of Poly-L-Lactide

Reference: Deng, M., Allan, J. M., Corbett, J. T., and Shalaby, S. W., **"Effects of Thermal History and Physical Aging on Thermal Properties of Poly-L-Lactide,"** *Synthetic Bioabsorbable Polymers for Implants, ASTM STP 1396*, C. M. Agrawal, J. E. Parr, and S. T. Lin, Eds., American Society for Testing and Materials, West Conshohocken, PA, 2000.

Abstract: Poly-L-lactide (PLL) represents a major bioabsorbable polymer used in implants. Depending on its thermal history, PLL can exhibit three discernible thermal transitions upon heating: glass transition, recrystallization, and melting. These transitions are pertinent to the polymer's short- and long-term performance. Accordingly, properties of medical devices made of PLL may be altered and optimized when subjected to different thermal environments. In the present study, differential scanning carlorometry was used to study effects of thermal treatment and physical aging on thermal properties of PLL. Heat treatment was conducted at three different temperatures. Physical aging was performed at room temperature for five different time intervals. Results indicate that glass transitions and level of crystallinity were affected significantly. The polymer crystallinity can be greatly increased by thermal treatment, which may ultimately improve its mechanical properties, as well as strength retention, and absorption profile. Relevance of these results to the physical events taking place during the treatment, and their impact on post-processing and property change of fabricated articles are discussed.

Keywords: poly-L-lactide, thermal property, crystallinity, DSC, bioabsorbable, physical aging, glass transition, thermal treatment, biomedical

Poly-L-lactide (PLL) is a semicrystalline polymer and it represents a major biomedical material [*1*]. PLL is biocompatible and degradable in biological environments and possesses good mechanical properties. As a result, the polymer has been used in biomedical implants such as fracture fixation devices. To better understand the polymer,

[1] Research scientist, manager of bioengineering, manager of pharmaceutical research, and director of research and development, respectively, Poly-Med, Inc., Research and Development Labs, 511 Westinghouse Road, Pendleton, SC 29670

meanwhile, considerable studies have been carried out on its processability, degradability, sterilization, and mechanical properties. However, the thermal properties of PLL have been relatively less explored. Thermal behavior is an important property that will greatly affect the heat-processing and performance of polymers. Depending on its thermal history, PLL can exhibit three discernible thermal transitions upon heating: glass transition, recrystallization, and melting. These transitions are pertinent to the polymer's short and long term performance both *in vitro* and *in vivo*. Accordingly, the properties of PLL may be altered or optimized when subjected to different thermal environments. This will provide us with more alternatives to design the properties of the medical devices made of this polymer by the predetermined thermal treatment.

Considering that thermal properties are some of the fundamental properties as they are closely related to the manufacturing, applications and performance of a polymer product, in the past, several papers have investigated the thermal properties and physical aging effects of poly-L-lactide (PLL) or poly(L-lactic acid) (PLLA) using widely available thermal analysis tools such as differential scanning carlorometry (DSC), thermogravimetric analysis (TGA), and dynamic mechanical thermal analysis (DMTA) [*2-5*]. However, a close look at these studies reveals no details on how the different thermal histories and physical aging may affect the ultimate thermal behavior of PLL, which are fundamentals to understand a polymer. This provides an incentive to pursue the present study.

In this investigation, DSC was used to study the effects of thermal history and physical aging on thermal properties of high molecular weight PLL. Heat treatment was conducted at three different temperatures, i.e., temperatures above melting (T_m), between recrystallization (T_c) and melting, and between glass transition (T_g) and recrystallization temperatures. This resulted in polymers having three types of thermal histories. For each type, physical aging was performed at room temperature for five different time intervals, which lasted for five decades. Results indicate that not only the glass transition temperature, but also level of crystallinity were affected significantly by different thermal treatment and physical aging. The polymer crystallinity can be greatly increased by eliminating the possibility of recrystallization, which may ultimately alter its mechanical properties, as well as strength retention, and absorption profiles in the biological environment. Relevance of these results to the physical events, taking place during the treatment, and their impact on post-processing and property change of the fabricated articles are addressed.

Materials and Methods

Granules of high molecular weight poly-L-lactide (PLL) prepared in this laboratory were used. The polymer was synthesized from L-lactide by ring-open polymerization. After synthesis, the polymer was kept under vacuum until use. Using chloroform as solvent, the inherent viscosity (IV) of the polymer was determined as 2.3 dl/g.

For thermal analysis, a Perkin Elmer DSC 6 differential scanning calorimeter was used to provide PLL with different thermal histories and to evaluate the thermal transitions of the polymer under controlled experimental conditions. Samples weighing about 5 mg were placed in an aluminum pan, compacted and scanned under nitrogen purge at constant scanning rates. The physical aging cycle was conducted on PLL at five time intervals, 0, 1, 10, 100, and 1000 minutes for three different thermal histories under nitrogen environment. That the longest aging time was chosen as 1000 minutes in this study was based on two assumptions: (1) this aging time would be long enough to see physical aging effects if any; (2) fast relaxation would occur within first few hours. These two assumptions hold for most polymers including PLL, the experimental material used in this investigation. All the experiments were performed in duplicate, i.e., two individual samples were used for the aging cycles.

To erase their original thermal histories acquired during polymerization and storage, all polymer samples were heated first to well above melting point, 210°C. The second step was to subject the polymer samples to different thermal histories as shown below. This was achieved by heating a sample from 20°C to a predetermined temperature T_t, held for 2 minutes at T_t, then cooled to 20°C to allow for physical aging. The T_t was above the material's glass transition temperature. The molten samples were not quick-quenched (e.g. using liquid nitrogen), but allowed to cool relatively slowly, which is more relevant to most industrial manufacturing processes. For all the collected DSC scans, the heating and cooling rates were 10 and 20°C/min, respectively. The detailed experimental design is described below.

Experiment 1: Step 1: heating from 20 to 210°C at 10°C/min; cooling from 210 to 20°C at 10°C/min;
Step 2: heating from 20 to 90°C at 10°C/min; holding for 2 minutes; cooling from 90 to 20°C at 20°C/min; holding for an aging time t_a;
Step 3: repeating second step for different aging time t_a.

Experiment 2: Step 1: heating from 20 to 210°C at 10°C/min; cooling from 210 to 20°C at 10°C/min;
Step 2: heating from 20 to 150°C at 10°C/min; holding for 2 minutes; cooling from 150 to 20°C at 10°C/min;
Step 3: heating from 20 to 90°C at 10°C/min; holding for 2 minutes; cooling from 90 to 20°C at 20°C/min; holding for an aging time t_a;
Step 4: repeating third step for different aging time t_a.

Experiment 3: Step 1: heating from 20 to 210°C at 10°C/min; cooling from 210 to 20°C at 10°C/min;
Step 2: heating from 20 to 210°C at 10°C/min; holding for 2 minutes; cooling from 210 to 20°C at 20°C/min; holding for an aging time t_a;
Step 3: repeating second step for different aging time t_a.

Results and Discussion

Figure 1 shows a typical DSC thermogram of the stored samples due to heating from 20 to 210°C at 10°C/min. This thermal behavior is typical for most of current PLL medical devices processed by injection and compression molding, extrusion and solvent casting. The thermogram clearly reveals three distinct thermal transition temperatures, T_g, T_c and T_m, associated with glass transition, recrystallization and melting. These transitions will have significance in predicting the performance and processing conditions for PLL. We can see from this thermogram that glass transition, recrystallization and melting take place at about 55°C, 105°C and 175°C, respectively. A glass transition temperature of 55°C will mean that PLL is a relatively stiff material at a temperature below 55°C (e.g. body temperature). Recrystallization near 105°C suggests that the crystallinity of PLL had a lower value than that revealed by the heat of fusion at melting. This was caused by inadequate crystallization upon cooling the polymer melt, which is due to mismatch between cooling and crystallization rates. Fast cooling rates lock the polymer chains into glass state before they could possibly form crystals. A peak melting point of about 175°C indicates that PLL should be melt-processed above this temperature for good properties. But the melting-processing temperature should be lower than the thermal degradation temperature as the lactide-containing polymers degrade rapidly above 260°C. Therefore, the experiments in the present study had been designed according to the recorded thermal characteristics of PLL, as illustrated in the experimental section, and the pertinent results are discussed below.

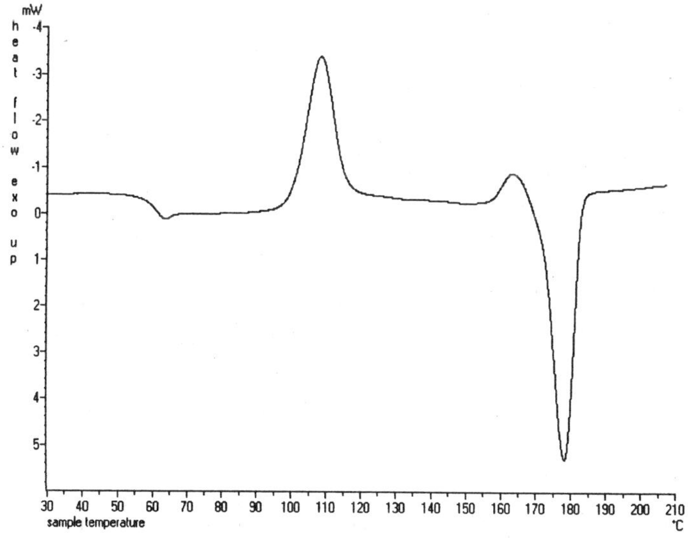

FIG. 1—*A typical DSC thermogram of PLL samples.*

Experiment 1 Results

Figure 2 illustrates typical experimentally-obtained DSC thermograms and their dependence on physical aging time. The temperature scans were from 20 to 90°C. The thermograms presented here cover the temperature range of 30 to 80°C to focus on glass transitions and the corresponding results revealed distinct glass transition for PLL in all scans. Table 1 outlines the data for the T_g and heat of relaxation (ΔH_g). The T_g's were calculated as the middle point of the glass transition region. It is understood from this table that the T_g's of the PLL are about 60°C and the physical aging time had little effect on T_g and ΔH_g, although their values tended to decrease a little. This is attributed to the facts: (a) relatively slow cooling rates of the polymer melt, which were slower than those of quick quenching, and (b) relatively short physical aging time periods. In other words, in order to see the differences in T_g and ΔH_g, we either have to quench or fast cool the polymer samples and/or let the physical aging process go beyond 1000 minutes. Additionally, the recrystallization and melting event were found not to be affected by physical aging for the examined physical aging time periods (the results were not presented here, although several experiments were conducted). The cooling rate of 20°C/min was slow enough to relax PLL (i.e., hardly to see physical aging effects), but it was still too fast for the polymer to fully crystallize (as was revealed by recrystallization peak during heating).

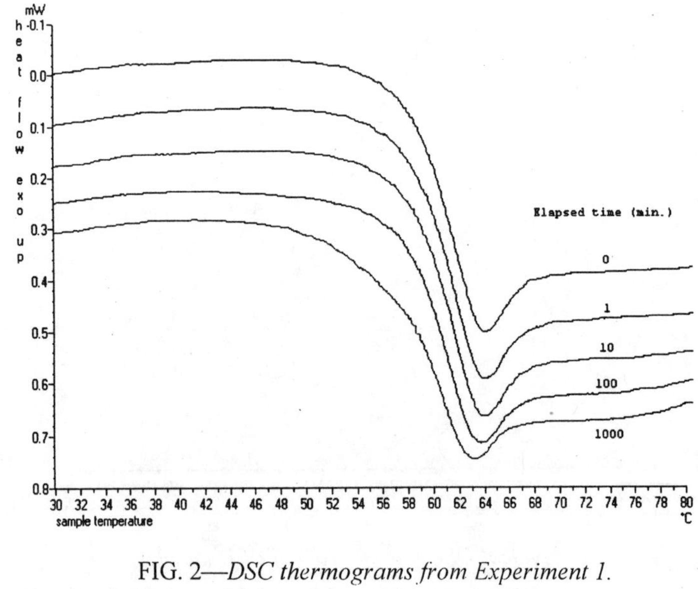

FIG. 2—*DSC thermograms from Experiment 1.*

Table 1—*Thermal data from Experiment 1.*

t_a, min.	T_g, °C	ΔH_g, J/g
0	60.2	1.05
1	60.1	1.20
10	60.3	1.15
100	60.0	1.19
1000	59.3	0.92

Experiment 2 Results

The purpose of this part of the study was to show how the crystallinity of PLL could be easily increased and the resulting effects on the glass transition temperature. In this experiment, the polymer samples were first heated to 150°C and then cooled to room temperature before starting the physical aging study. The heating scheme is illustrated in Figure 3, which depicts a strong recrystallization exotherm. The purpose of this step was to allow recrystallization to occur in order to increase the degree of crystallinity. Accordingly, the thermogram (Figure 4) of the resulting specimen of PLL showed no recrystallization events before melting, which is distinctly different than Figure 1.

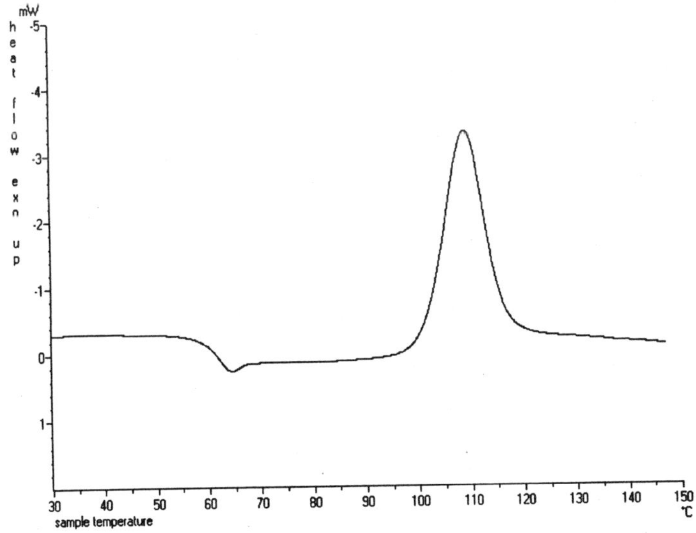

FIG. 3—*DSC thermogram showing heating PLL samples to 150°C.*

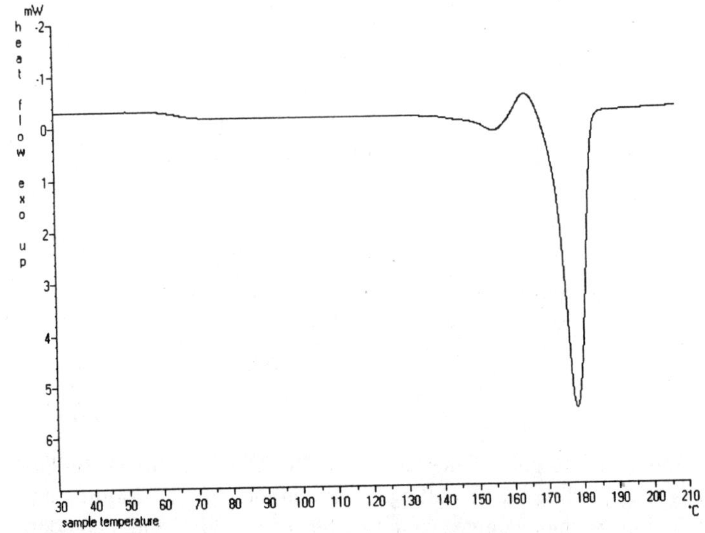

FIG. 4—*Heating PLL samples to 210°C after thermal treatment.*

Figure 5 shows the dependence of glass transition on physical aging. It is obvious that the DSC thermograms in Figure 5 are significantly different than those in Figure 2. Table 2 presents the T_g of PLL under the conditions of Experimental 2. It can be seen from this table that the glass transition temperatures here are about 65°C, which are significantly higher than those shown in Table 1. It is reasonable to suggest that the higher T_g's are due to an increase of about 40% in percent crystallinity. The increase in crystallinity would have two consequences. First, in a semi-crystalline polymer, crystals function as physical cross-links, which interfere with the segmental chain motion. Second, the amorphous phase is reduced due to the increase in the crystalline phase contribution to a unit volume. This will, in turn, decrease the free volume of the polymer. As a result, the T_g's of PLL were extended to higher temperature. On the other hand, Table 2 shows that physical aging had little effect on T_g when aging time is at or lower than 100 min. However, significantly higher T_g was observed when aging time reached 1000 min. ΔH_g is too small to be measured. It was also found that melting transitions were not effected by physical aging and the increase in crystallinity.

It can be inferred from the above results that an increase in crystallinity would lead to higher mechanical strength and longer degradation time both *in vitro* and *in vivo* for PLL materials. Accordingly, heat-treated or annealed medical devices made of PLL would have a better mechanical performance than untreated ones. This can be explained further. For a semi-crystalline polymer, its strength and modulus are primarily dependent on percentage of crystalline phase. During the hydrolysis degradation of this polymer, the amorphous phase is first attacked. On the other hand, most of crystalline phase is hardly affected until the amorphous phase is broken down and water diffuses into the polymer. So the PLL with higher crystallinity will last longer and hold more load during implantation. This is important for PLL as a load-bearing implant. To a device manufacturer, the results presented here also suggest a simple way to improve or design mechanical properties of PLL-based medical devices so that their performance in a biological environment can be optimized.

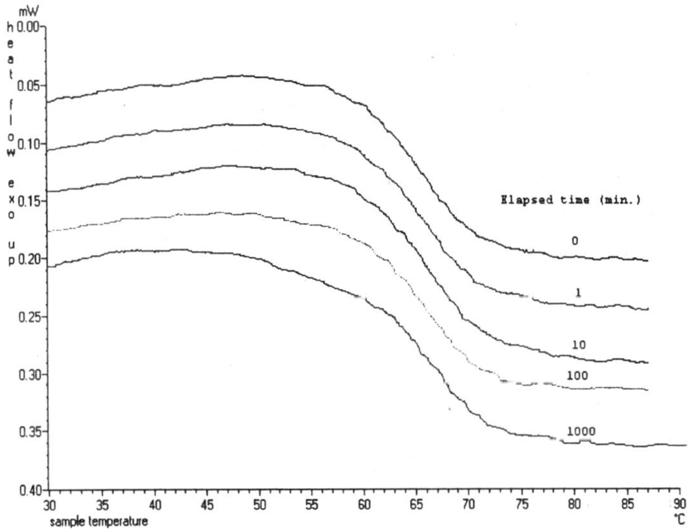

FIG. 5—*DSC thermograms from Experiment 2.*

Table 2—*Thermal data from Experiment 2.*

ta, min.	T_g, °C	ΔH_g, J/g
0	64.7	N/A
1	65.6	N/A
10	65.9	N/A
100	65.5	N/A
1000	67.6	N/A

Experiment 3 Results

If heating PLL to 90°C can fully release internal stresses and relax molecular chains within amorphous phase, then test samples from Experiment 3 would display few differences than those from Experiment 2. Toward addressing this question the DSC study as defined in Experiment 3 was pursued, and the effects of physical aging time on thermal transitions are illustrated in Figure 6. Figure 7 shows an enlargement of the glass transition area, which is very similar to those in Figure 2 for the aging time periods up to 100 minutes. At t_a = 1000 minutes, the glass transition is much different, which is yet to be explained. Table 3 outlines the thermal properties for PLL. It is apparent from the data presented in the table that these properties were hardly affected by physical aging from periods of 100 minutes or less. However, at t_a = 1000 minutes, relatively low T_g, T_c and ΔH_m were observed, but T_m was not effected. The experimental results also indicated that there were distinct recrystallization events. Considering this fact, the polymer should have a much lower crystallinity than that calculated from melting endotherm. And the mechanical properties of such PLL devices should not be as good as those from Experiment 2.

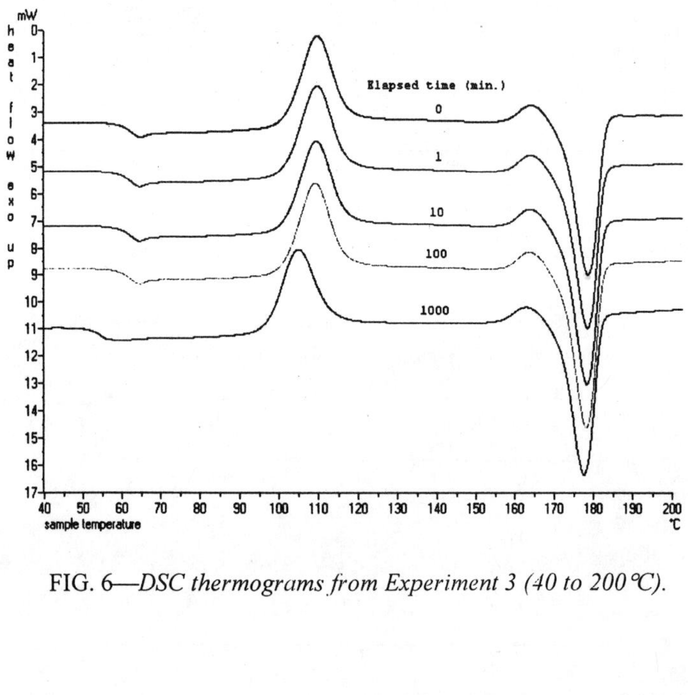

FIG. 6—*DSC thermograms from Experiment 3 (40 to 200°C).*

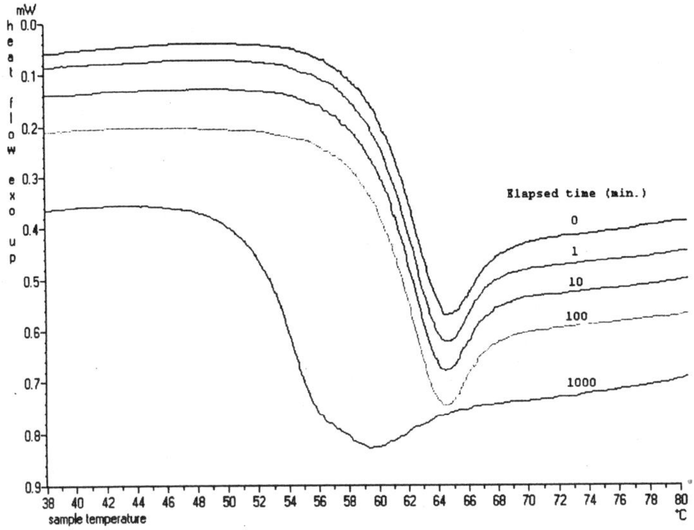

FIG. 7—*DSC thermograms from Experiment 3 (38 to 80°C).*

Table 3—*Thermal data from Experiment 3.*

t_a, min.	T_g, °C	ΔH_g, J/g	T_c, °C	ΔH_c, J/g	ΔH_m, J/g	T_m, °C
0	61.2	1.37	109.6	-35.4	54.2	178.6
1	60.8	1.16	109.5	-35.0	54.0	178.4
10	61.0	0.94	109.5	-36.2	53.4	178.3
100	60.9	0.93	109.1	-36.5	54.3	178.1
1000	54.4	1.05	105.3	-35.2	51.9	177.7

Conclusions

The study showed that the physical aging and heat treatments (or annealing) do affect the thermal properties and crystallinity of PLL. Understanding these effects would definitely contribute to the development of PLL-based medical devices with improved performance. This study also suggests a simple method to increase the crystallinity of

PLL so that the mechanical performance of the polymer can be improved and designed. This is particularly important for load-bearing implants. Although several other methods such as slow cooling, orientation and high pressure application can be used to increase crystallinity, they may sometimes be impractical economically for device manufacturers.

References

[1] Shalaby, S. W., *Biomedical Polymers: Designed-to-Degrade Systems*, Chapter 1, Hanser/Gardner Publications, Inc., Cincinnati, Ohio, USA, 1994.

[2] Engelberg, I. and Kohn, J. "Physico-Mechanical Properties of Degradable Polymers Used in Medical Applications: a Comparative Study," *Biomaterials*, Vol 12, April, 1991 pp. 292-304.

[3] Celli, A. and Scandola, M. "Thermal Properties and Physical Ageing of Poly(L-Lactic Acid)," *Polymer*, Vol 33, No 13, 1992, pp. 2699-2703.

[4] Cai, H., Dave, V., Gross, R. A., and MaCarthy, S. P., "Effects of Physical Aging, Crystallinity, and Orientation on the Enzymatic Degradation of Poly(Lactic Acid)," *Journal of Polymer Science: Part B: Polymer Physics*, Vol. 34, 1996, pp. 2701-2708.

[5] Gogolewski, S. and Mainil-Varlet, P., "The Effect of Thermal Treatment on Sterility, Molecular and Mechanical Properties of Various Polylactides: I. Poly(L-Lactide)," *Biomaterials*, Vol. 17, No. 15, 1996, pp. 523-528.

Nick L. Jones,[1] John J. Cooper,[2] Russell D. Waters,[2] and David F. Williams[1]

Resorption Profile and Biological Response of Calcium Phosphate filled PLLA and PHB7V

Reference: Jones, N. L., Cooper, J. J., Waters, R. D., and Williams, D. F., **"Resorption Profile and Biological Response of Calcium Phosphate filled PLLA and PHB7V,"** *Synthetic Bioabsorbable Polymers for Implants, ASTM STP 1396*, C. M. Agrawal, J. E. Parr, and S. T. Lin, Eds., American Society for Testing and Materials, West Conshohocken, PA, 2000.

Abstract: A study was performed to assess the effects of tri-calcium phosphate filler on the tissue response, mechanical properties and degradation characteristics of injection moulded poly L-lactide (PLLA) and poly-hydroxybutyrate co valerate (7 mole % valerate) (PHB7V).

Test pieces for mechanical evaluation were prepared according to ASTM and British Standards. These were aged both *in vitro*, using a phosphate buffered saline solution (PBS) at pH 7.4 and 37°C and *in vivo*, subcutaneously using Dutch rabbits. Tensile strength of the materials was monitored, together with molecular weight (Mw) of the polymer as determined by gel permeation chromatography (GPC). The host response to intraosseous implants placed transcortically in the femurs of New Zealand rabbits, was assessed using an undecalcified, unstained, polarised light technique on resin embedded and polished sections.

The materials had good biocompatibility. The bone response to the polymers and composites was very similar. Histology showed that new bone was formed at the defect site, which grew up to the material surface and remodelled into new physiological bone tissue. The rate of degradation of the poly-L-lactide and it's composite with tri-calcium phosphate as assessed by tensile strength and Mw was found to be consistent with the rate for bone healing. Poly-hydroxybutyrate co valerate and its composite with tri-calcium phosphate degraded more slowly.

Keywords: PLLA, PHB, composite, degradation, resorption

---

[1]Student and Professor respectively, Department of Clinical Engineering, University of Liverpool, Duncan Building, Royal Liverpool University Hospital, Liverpool, L69 3BX. United Kingdom.

[2]Technical Research Director and Operations Director respectively, Biocomposites Ltd, Etruscan Street, Etruria, Stoke-on-Trent, ST1 5PQ. United Kingdom.

Introduction

Many studies have shown that highly rigid fixation of bone fragments prevents complete healing, since much of the load that is normally carried by the bone is transferred across the fracture site by the implant (stress shielding effect). This stress shielded area is susceptible to refracture if the implant is removed. Conversely, gross motion at the fracture site due to poor fixation or the use of materials with a modulus lower than that of bone can also result in incomplete healing or non-union.

Bioresorbable polymers are a class of materials that are now being used in a wide range of medical applications. These include soft tissue support such as sutures and wound care patches and hard tissue repair and fixation such as plates, screws and pins. The rate of healing of bone and the establishment of viable haversian systems is about six weeks in man [*1*] and hence materials for fracture support should maintain adequate strength throughout this time frame. Resorbable polymers are also being investigated for controlled release drug delivery [*2*] and as a resorbable scaffold to support cell implantation in tissue engineering applications [*3*].

Most synthetic biodegradable polymers including poly glycolic acid (PGA), poly lactic acid (PLA) and poly hydroxybutyric acid (PHB) are polyesters which degrade through hydrolysis of the ester bond in the polymer backbone. The degradation products are the simple acid repeat units which can be safely metabolised by the body. The degradation rate depends upon the polymers hydrophilic/hydrophobic nature together with the Mw and degree of crystallinity[*4*]. In this group the most polar or hydrophilic is PGA and this resorbs the fastest. PHB is the most hydrophobic and this resorbs the slowest. Poly lactides are intermediate in this respect and their rate of degradation and loss of strength can be consistent with the rate of healing of bone. This allows the healing bone to gradually restore its physiological load bearing function.

These polymers can be processed by techniques such as injection moulding which is a very efficient and cost-effective method of producing complex net-shaped components.

In order to improve the potential of these materials for many orthopaedic and maxillofacial applications, bioceramic fillers can be introduced to give biocomposite materials with properties more appropriate to the clinical need than the polymers, or copolymers alone[*5*]. The addition of certain bioactive fillers, such as hydroxyapatite (HAp) or tri-calcium phosphate (TCP), to a resorbable polymer can confer a number of advantages. Increasing levels of fillers to polymers result in increasing modulus, such that modulus matching to bone becomes possible [*6*]. The use of HAp or TCP which are osteoconductive materials, could help to provide an environment for new bone in-growth as the polymeric component resorbs. These materials can have a radio-density similar to bone and this will help to enable the implant to be imaged by standard X-ray techniques. (Pure polymeric components are invisible to X-rays).

A number of previous studies [*7, 8*] have reported a late foreign body reaction and weeping sinus associated with PLA and PGA. It was suggested that a lowering of pH in the vicinity of the implant could be a factor. Li et al [*9*] have described a mechanism of autocatalytic degradation for the poly(α- hydroxy) acids whereby the acidic degradation products build up within the polymer faster than they can diffuse away. This low pH environment accelerates the rate of further degradation. A technique to control the pH in the vicinity of biodegradable polymeric implants has been described by Van Der Meer et al [*10*] and Agrawal et al [*11*]. This involves the addition of certain fillers to biodegradable polymers to react with and neutralise the acidic byproducts of hydrolysis.

The results of an *in vitro* and *in vivo* degradation study and intraosseous tissue response of PLLA, PHB7V, PLLA10%TCP and PHB7V10%TCP are described.

Materials and Methods

Poly-hydroxybutyrate 7% valerate copolymer (PHB7V) was a commercially available material, BIOPOL® [3]. Its Mw was reported as 550 000 and melting point as 150°C. Poly(L)Lactide (PLLA) was a medical grade material, PURASORB® [4]. Its Mw was reported as 360 000 and melting point as 190°C. In the as-moulded condition, both polymers are essentially amorphous.

The calcium phosphate, ALLOGRAN-R™ [5], was prepared from a stoichiometric mixture of dicalcium phosphate and lime to give beta tri-calcium orthophosphate which conformed to Standard Specification for Beta-Tri-Calcium Phosphate for Surgical Implantation, ASTM F1088-87. The only phase detected by X-ray Diffraction analysis (XRD) was whitlockite. The material consisted of polycrystalline aggregates having a mean agglomerate size of 100 - 200 microns and a crystal size of 1 - 2 microns.

The polymers were injection moulded according to the suppliers recommendations using a MANUMOLD [6] 77/30 Screw Injection Moulding Machine. For the PHB7V and its composite, temperatures of 130°C and 150°C for the barrel and nozzle respectively were used. For the PLLA and its composite, the corresponding temperatures were 180°C and 190°C. A 10 vol.% fill composition of each polymer with TCP was prepared using densities of TCP = 3.14g/cc, PLLA = 1.24 g/cc and PHB7V = 1.25 g/cc, in order to calculate the weight proportions of each component.

A typical scanning electron microscope image (SEM) showing a fracture surface of the polymer composite as-moulded is shown in Figure 1.

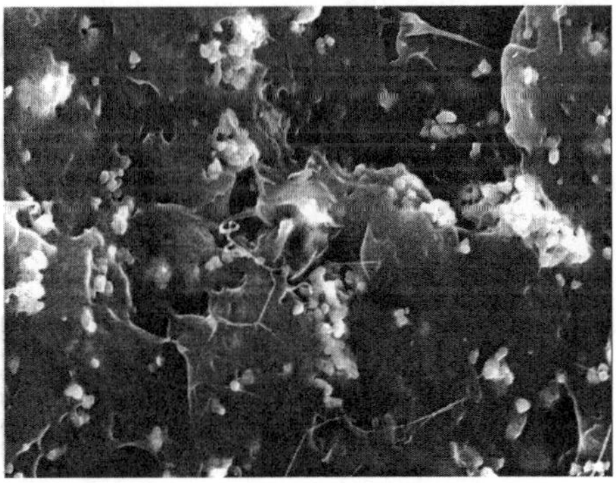

20μm

Figure 1 Polymer Composite as Moulded

[3]Zeneca, Cleveland, United Kingdom.
[4]Purac Biochem bv, Gorinchem, Holland.
[5]Biocomposites Ltd, Stoke on Trent, Staffordshire, United Kingdom.
[6]Manumould, Luton, Bedfordshire, United Kingdom.

Individual TCP crystallites can be seen, together with polycrystalline agglomerates. The high shear conditions which exist during the injection moulding process have caused some fragmentation of the original TCP particles. Examination of a number of sections through moulded pieces has shown a uniform distribution of the filler particles in the polymer matrix.

Test pieces were prepared to Test Method for Tensile Properties of Plastics, ASTM D638 and Determination of Tensile Properties, Test Conditions for Moulding and Extrusion Plastics, BS2782, Part 3.

In vitro testing was performed in PBS pH 7.4 at 37°C. The samples were put into glass screw top bottles containing physiologic soaking solution which consisted of PBS at pH = 7.4. The solution: specimen mass ratio was approximately 100:1. The bottles containing the samples were then put into a heated air oven where the temperature was maintained at 37 ± 2°C for the duration of the experiment. The pH of the solution was monitored (initially daily and then weekly) and the solution replaced with fresh PBS when deemed necessary to maintain the pH in the range 7.4 ± 0.2. At the selected time periods the bottles were removed from the oven and allowed to cool to room temperature (22 ± 2°C). The samples were removed from the solution and the surface was dried with a paper towel. The samples were then dried at 37°C for 24 hours prior to testing. Five samples per time period were tested using a Nene Mechanical Testing Machine, at a loading rate of 5 mm/min.

For *in vivo* testing, the smaller "dog-bone" shaped tensile test specimens were used. They were sterilised by gamma irradiation to 2.5Mrad and then implanted subcutaneously, five samples per animal, in the dorso lumbar region using fully mature Dutch rabbits weighing between 2.5 and 3.0 kg. At the selected time periods the animals were sacrificed and the implants retrieved. These were carefully cleaned of soft tissue, and dried at 37°C for twenty four hours prior to testing. These smaller specimens were tested using a loading rate of 1 mm/min.

Intraosseous implantation for histological examination was performed using fully mature New Zealand white rabbits weighing between 3.5 and 6.0 kg. The implants were injection moulded pins of 2.5 mm diameter, which were subsequently cut to 8 - 10 mm length. They were ultrasonically cleaned, dried and irradiated prior to implantation. Up to five samples per femur spaced at approximately 8 mm intervals were press-fit inserted transcortically. Animals were sacrificed for histological evaluation at time periods of 6, 8, 12, 16, 20, 24 and 32 weeks for PLLA and PLLA/TCP and 12, 24, 36 and 52 weeks for PHB7V and PHB7V/TCP. All procedures were performed to strict national guidelines. Due to the known slower degradation rate of PHBV compared to PLLA, longer time periods for all tests were chosen.

Mechanical Measurements

In vitro and *in vivo* samples were removed at each time period, washed in distilled water, blotted with filter paper to remove excess water and then dried at 37°C for 24 hrs prior to testing. Five samples were tested for each condition and at each time period.

Molecular Weight

Degradation of the polymer is accompanied by a reduction in its Mw. The average Mw of the polymer was determined at the selected time periods by size exclusion chromatography (SEC). This technique, which is also known as gel permeation chromatography (GPC), involves dissolving the polymer in a suitable solvent and passing this through a microporous gel-filled column. The residence time of the polymer in the column depends upon its Mw. Elution of the polymer from the column is monitored by a refractive index detector. The solvent used was chloroform and the polymer concentration 0.5% w/v. The analyses were performed at ambient temperature with a flow rate of 1.0 ml/min. Polystyrene was used as a Mw calibration standard.

Histology

Explantation of the samples and surrounding bony tissue was undertaken at the selected time periods. Tissue response to the implants was assessed using an un-decalcified method. After sacrifice the rabbits femurs were sectioned, using a low speed saw, into smaller tissue blocks prior to initiating histological processing. Dehydration was accomplished using methanol water mixtures with an ascending concentration to 100% absolute methanol. Embedding was performed using methylmethacrylate infiltration, followed by polymerisation. Sections were taken using an ISOMET™ [7] low speed saw and these were carefully polished before mounting onto PERSPEX® [8] slides. Final polishing was undertaken with increasingly finer diamond grit. Five samples per material per time period were used and histological evaluation was undertaken on unstained sections using polarisation microscopy and a Zeiss fully automatic photo-microscope

Results and Discussion

Mechanical Properties

The results of tensile testing of PLLA and PLLA/TCP aged *in vitro* are shown in Figure 2a. Tensile strength is recorded for each time period. The values represent mean ± SD of five samples. The effect of the 10% volume TCP filler is to reduce the initial tensile strength from approximately 65MPa to 46MPa. For the PLLA, the strength is maintained for a time period of sixteen weeks, at which point it starts to fall and by forty weeks no measurable strength remains.

For the composite, the initial strength is 46MPa and is maintained to within 90% of this initial value for a time period of twenty four to twenty six weeks. From this point, the strength falls more rapidly to a point of no measurable strength at again forty weeks.

[7]Buehler Ltd, Coventry, United Kingdom.
[8]Plexiglass, Visijor Plastics Ltd, Warrington, United Kingdom.

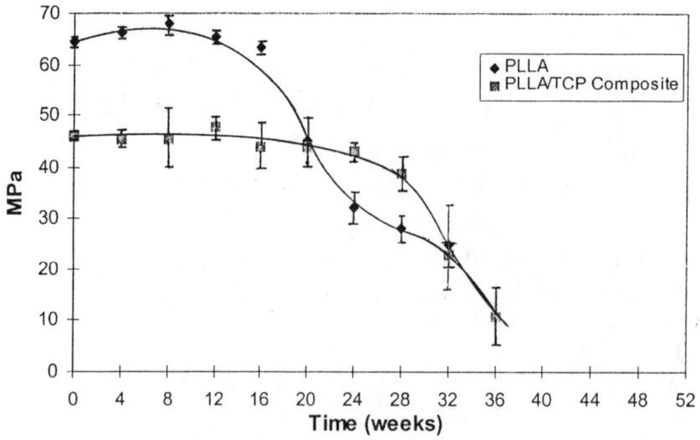

Figure 2a Tensile Strength Vs Time In Vitro

For PLLA and PLLA/TCP *in vivo*, Figure 2b, a similar trend is observed, but over a shorter time frame. The PLLA has an initial strength of 67MPa which falls gently to 60MPa at eight weeks, where the rate of fall increases giving a value at twenty weeks of 17MPa. The composite has an initial value of 48MPa which shows a gradual fall to 42MPa over sixteen weeks, from which point the rate of fall increases to give a value of 32MPa at the final, twenty week, time point. All of the implants were easily retrieved from the surrounding soft tissue, and there was no indication of any adverse tissue response.

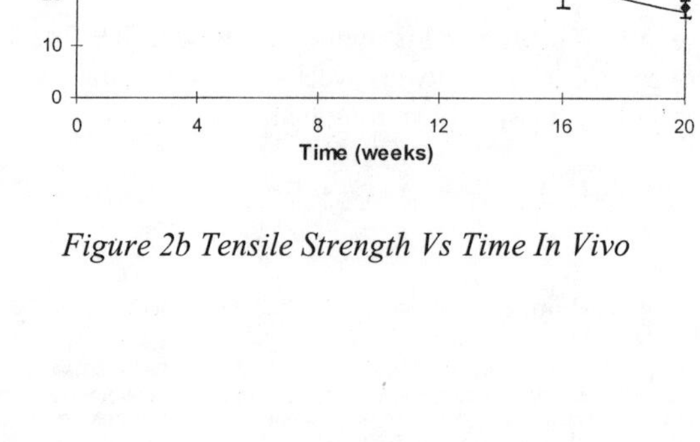

Figure 2b Tensile Strength Vs Time In Vivo

Figure 3a shows the tensile strength for PHB7V and PHB7V/TCP, *in vitro*. The initial strength values are approximately half those for the equivalent PLLA and PLLA/TCP. The PHB7V gives a value of 34MPa which appears to increase to 36MPa at four months and then gradually decreases to a value of 18MPa at the final, thirty month, time point.

The composite again starts lower at 28MPa appearing to increase slightly to 29MPa at four months and then slowly falling to 20MPa at the final, thirty month, time point.

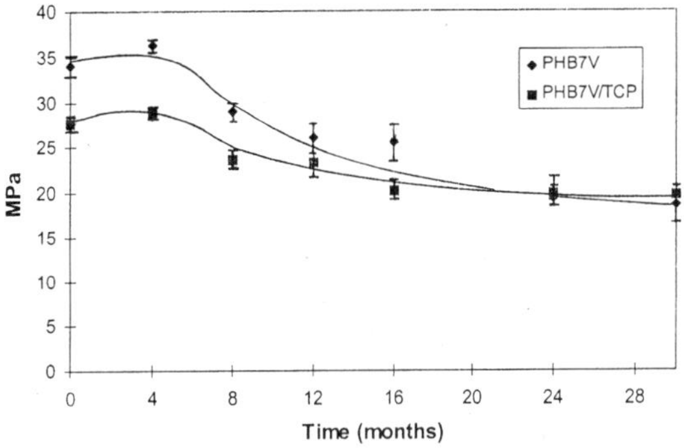

Figure 3a Tensile Strength Vs Time In Vitro

A very similar trend is observed *in vivo*, Figure 3b, but again over a shorter time frame. The initial strength values are 34MPa and 28MPa for PHB7V and PHB7V/TCP respectively, with both showing a barely significant increase at the three month time point. From this point, the strength of both falls continuously to give values at the final fifteen month time point of 4MPa for the polymer and no measurable strength for the composite.

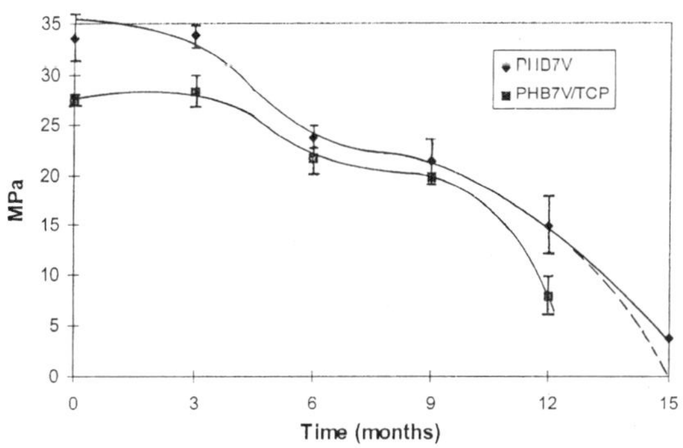

Figure 3b Tensile Strength Vs Time In Vivo

During the injection moulding process, molten polymer is forced into a steel cavity where it quickly cools and solidifies. This can result in "frozen-in" stresses due to uneven cooling. When the polymer specimens are put into an aqueous environment, water will diffuse into the sample to begin the process of hydrolysis. The authors suggest that this mechanism may amount to a stress-relief annealing process and account for the observed small increase in tensile strength at the early time periods.

Molecular Weight

Mw as determined by GPC is shown in Figures 4 and 5. For the polymers and the composites, both *in vitro* and *in vivo*, Mw is seen to fall steadily from time zero with a rate of fall which reduces with increasing time. The time-zero values of Mw are lower for the *in vivo* samples than the corresponding *in vitro* samples and this is maintained for the duration of the experiment. The gamma rays used to sterilise all the *in vivo* samples prior to implantation have a high energy sufficient to cause scission of the polymer chains thus lowering its Mw. Also, the body temperature of the rabbit at 39°C is slightly higher than the *in vitro* test temperature of 37°C.

The rate of reduction of Mw is greater for the PLLA than for the PHB7V by approximately a factor of x 4. This is in general agreement with data presented by Gogolewski et al [*12*], and can be accounted for by the more hydrophobic nature of the PHB/V materials.

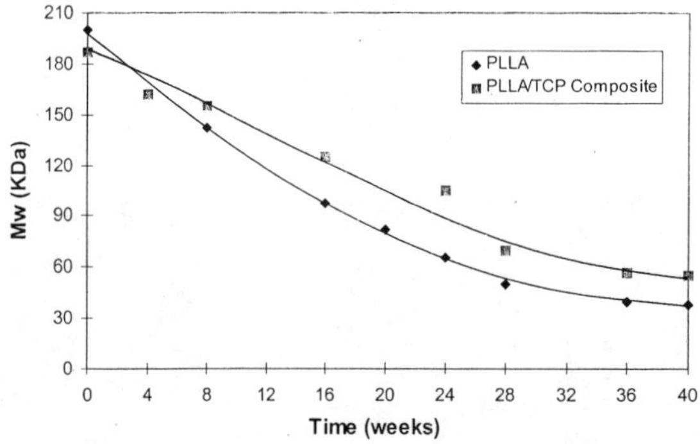

Figure 4a Molecular Weight (Mw) Vs Time in Vitro

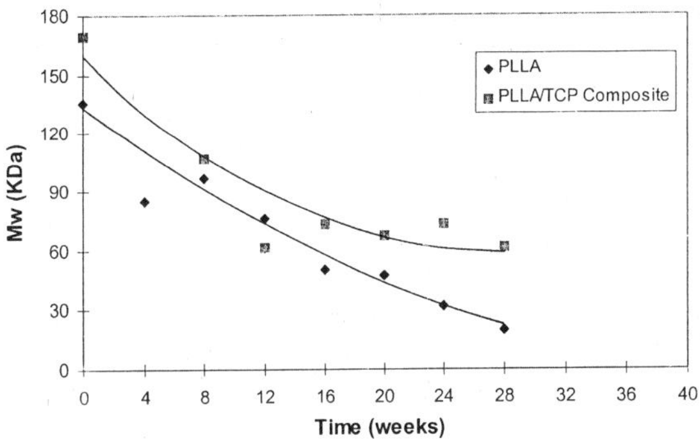

Figure 4b Molecular Weight (Mw) Vs Time in Vivo

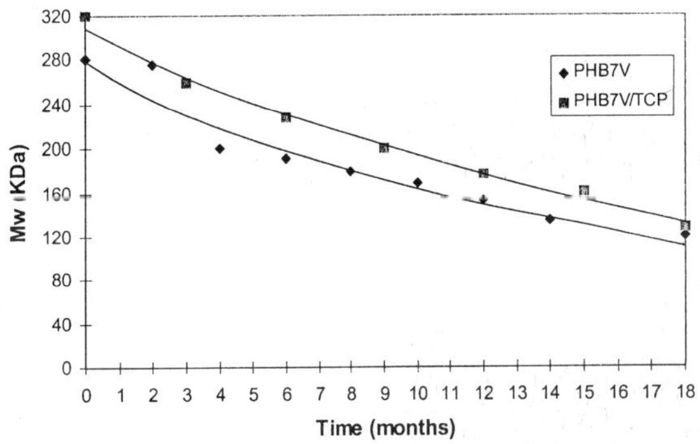

Figure 5a Molecular Weight (Mw) Vs Time In Vitro

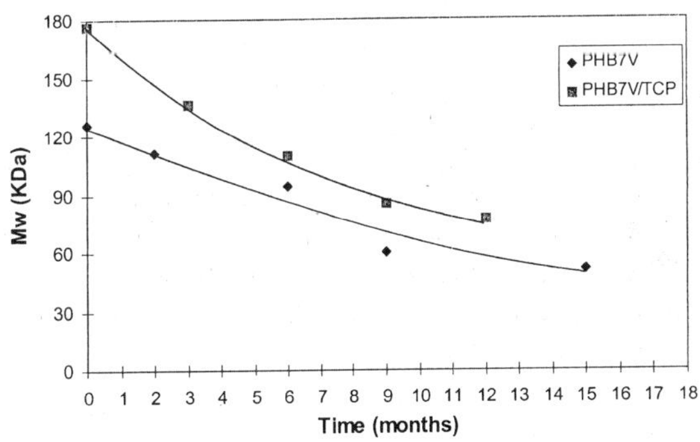

Figure 5b Molecular Weight (Mw) Vs Time In Vivo

It can be seen that, overall, the values of Mw are lower for the polymer than the corresponding composite. It is not clear why this should be the case and further work will be necessary to confirm, or otherwise, this result and elucidate the mechanism.

Histology

Figure 6 shows a section of the PLLA implant at sixteen weeks. Considerable swelling of the material both within the medullary cavity and outside the cortical rim is clearly evident. Within the cortical rim the material is constrained. This will result in a compressive stress field in this region. New bone tissue has formed from both the periosteal and endosteal aspects of the original cortical bone. Bone trabeculae originating from the opposite endosteal region, and covering the bottom of the implant, is also apparent. By this sixteen week period, the implant has been encapsulated by bone which has remodelled into what appears to be mature healthy bone. The cracks which are visible within the polymer could be an artefact of the section preparation conditions.

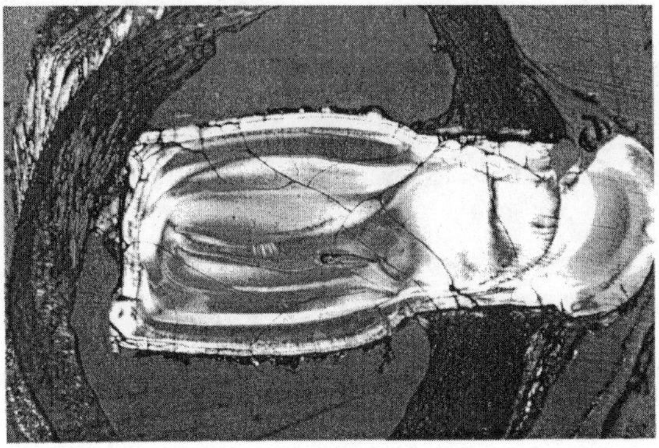

Figure 6 PLLA sixteen weeks X 1

A higher magnification view of the interface between bone and implant taken at thirty two weeks (Figure 7), shows a very close adaptation and contouring of both these surfaces with new bone forming to the contours of the polymer

Figure 8 shows a section of the PLLA/TCP implant at six weeks. Swelling of the material within the medullary cavity and outside the cortical rim is again clearly evident. Where the implant passes through the cortical rim a close adaptation between bone and implant is apparent. Even at this early time period new bone tissue is forming both endosteally and periosteally, while new bone trabeculae are originating at the endosteal aspect of the inner cortex and contacting the end of the implant.

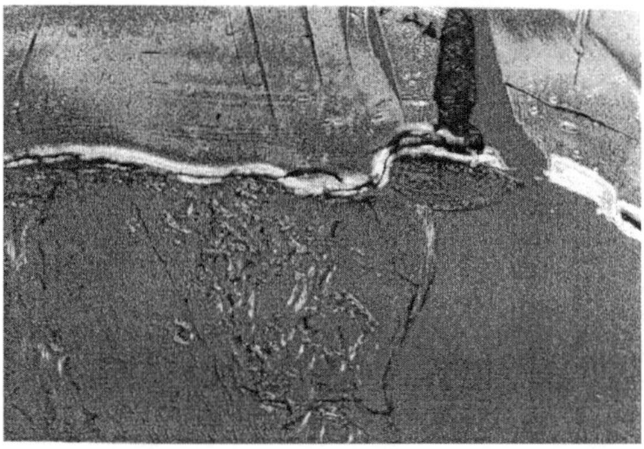

Figure 7 PLLA - bone interface at thirty two weeks X 6.3

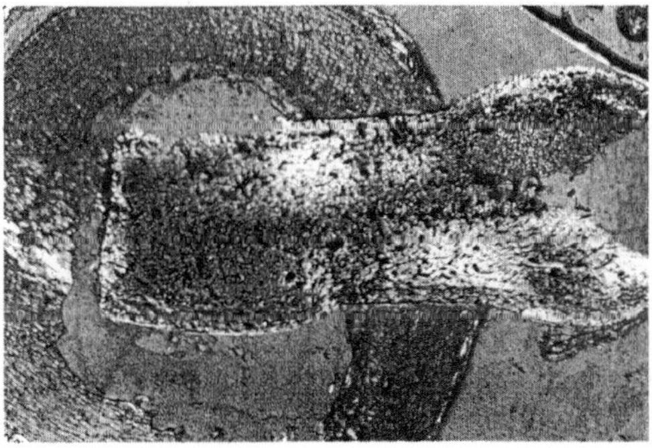

Figure 8 PLLA/TCP six weeks X 1

At thirty two weeks, Figure 9, the implant is seen to be fragmenting. Small fragments are encapsulated in healthy new bone, which has formed in close adaptation to the implant surface.

The bone response to PHB7V and PHB7V/TCP is similar to that shown for PLLA and PLLA/TCP. New healthy bone grows up to and over the surface of the implant, both periosteally and endosteally and close adaptation between bone and implant is seen. This polymer, however, shows very little swelling and no apparent fragmentation, even at the fifty two week time period, Figure 10.

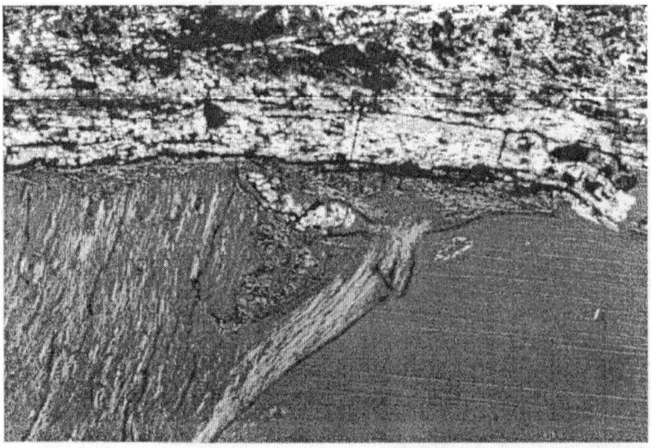

Figure 9 PLLA/TCP-bone interface at thirty two weeks X 6.3

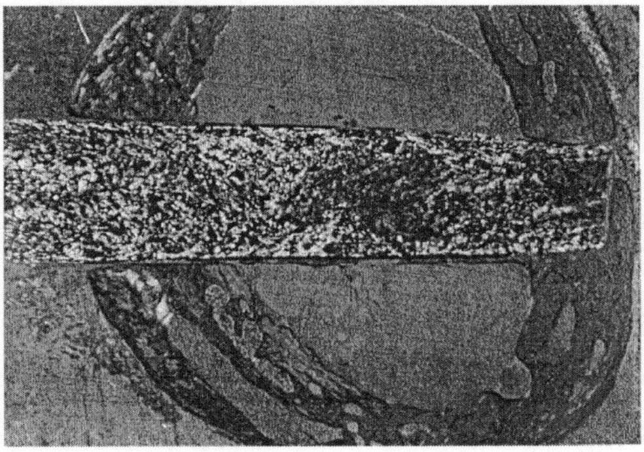

Figure 10 PHB7V/TCP fifty two weeks X 1

Conclusions

The tissue response, both intraosseous and intramuscular, of all four materials tested to the time periods indicated was good, with no signs of any inflammatory or adverse effects.

The PHB7V and its composite with TCP gave a rate of degradation, as assessed by both tensile strength and Mw, approximately four times slower than the corresponding PLLA and PLLA/TCP.

The rate of degradation *in vivo* for all four materials was approximately double the rate *in vitro*. However, since all *in vivo* samples were sterilised by gamma irradiation and thus had a lower initial Mw than the unirradiated *in vitro* samples, direct comparison is impossible. For comparative work, all samples that are tested *in vitro* should be sterilised by the method appropriate for *in vivo* samples.

The addition of the 10%volTCP filler to PLLA has given a biocomposite material having an extended strength and Mw retention period both *in vitro* and *in vivo*. It is proposed that the characteristics of this type of biocomposite material make them suitable candidates for improved devices for orthopaedic applications.

Acknowledgement

Thanks go to Dr J Hunt, Dr K Albastany and Dr P Doherty, University of Liverpool for the implantation and histology work and to the Engineering and Physical Sciences Research Council, London, United Kingdom, for financial support for this study.

References

[1] Simmons, D. J., and Urist, M. R. (Ed.), "Fracture Healing, Fundamental and Clinical Bone Physiology," J B Lippencott Co Philadelphia, 1980, pp. 283-330.

[2] Kopecek, J., "Controlled Biodegradation of Polymers - A Key to Drug Delivery Systems," *Biomaterials,* 1984, Vol. 5, pp. 19-25.

[3] Lu, L., and Mikos, A. G., "The Importance of New Processing Techniques in Tissue Engineering," *Mat. Res. Soc. Bull.,* 1996, Vol. 21, No. 11, November, pp. 28-32.

[4] Williams, D. F., "Mechanisms of Biodegradation of Implantable Polymers," *Clinical Materials*, 1992, Vol. 10, pp. 9-12.

[5] Boeree, N. R., Dove, J., Cooper, J. J., Knowles, J., and Hasting, G. W., "Development of a Degradable Composite for Orthopaedic Use: Mechanical Evaluation of a Hydroxyapatite-Polyhydroxybutyrate Composite Material," *Biomaterials*, 1993, Vol. 14, No.10, pp. 793-796.

[6] Doyle, C., Tanner, E. T., and Bonfield, W., "*In Vitro* and *In Vivo* Evaluation of polyhydroxybutyrate and polyhydroxybutyrate Reinforced with Hydroxyapatite," *Biomaterials,* 1991, Vol. 12, November, pp. 841-847

[7] Böstman, O. M., and Pihlajamäki, H. K., "Late Foreign-Body Reaction to an Intraosseous Bioabsorbable Polylactic Acid Screw," *Journal of Bone and Joint Surgery,* 1998, Vol. 80A, No.12, pp. 1791-1794.

[8] Bergsma, J. E., de Bruijn, W. C., Rozema, F. R., Bos, R. R., and Boering, G., "Late Degradation Tissue Response to Poly(L-Lactide) Bone Plates and Screws," *Biomaterials*, 1995, Vol. 16, pp. 25-31.

[9] Li, S., Garreau, H., and Vert, M., "Structure-Property Relationships in the Case of the Degradation of Massive Poly(∝-hydroxy)acids in Aqueous Media. Part 3. Influence of the Morphology of Poly(L-Lactic) Acid," *J. Mater. Sci. Mater. Med.,* 1990, Vol. 1, pp 198-206

[10] Van Der Meer, S. A. T., Wijn, J. R., and Wolke, J. G. C., "The Influence of Basic Filler Materials on the Degradation of Amorphous D- and L-Lactide Copolymer," *J Mater. Sci. Mater. Med.,* 1996, Vol. 7, pp. 359-361

[11] Agrawal, C. M., Fan, M., Zhu, C., and Athanasiou, K. A., "A New Technique to Control the pH in the Vicinity of Biodegradable Implants," *Fifth World Biomaterials Congress, Toronto Canada,* 1996.

[12] Gogolewski, S., Jovanovic, M., Perren, S. M., Dillon, J. G., and Hughes, M. K., "Tissue Response and *In Vivo* Degradation of Selected Polyhydroxyacids," *J. Bio. Mats. Res.,* 1993, Vol. 27, pp. 1135-1148

Dietmar W. Hutmacher,[1] Axel Kirsch,[2] Karl L. Ackermann,[2] Harald Liedtke,[3] and Markus B. Hürzeler[4]

The Clinical Evaluation of a Bioresorbable Minipin

Reference: Hutmacher, D. W., Kirsch, A., Ackermann, K. L., Liedtke, H., and Hürzeler, M. B., **"The Clinical Evaluation of a Bioresorbable Minipin,"** *Synthetic Bioabsorbable Polymers for Implants, STP 1396,* C. M. Agrawal, J. E. Parr, and S. T. Lin, Eds., American Society for Testing and Materials, West Conshohocken, PA, 2000.

Abstract: The gradual shift from nonresorbable membranes to biodegradable and bioresorbable membranes represents one of the most significant trends in guided tissue regeneration (GTR) and guided bone regeneration (GBR) research. The clinical benefits of biodegradable and bioresorbable membranes that have the capacity to integrate with surrounding soft and hard tissues are a result of a more mechanically stable and therefore predictable wound healing environment. This biomechanical stability can be further enhanced by the stabilization of the physical barrier construct using additional fixation devices. Therefore, bioresorbable minipins have been desigened and fabricated. The minipins are made of poly (L-lactid-co-D, L-lactid) in a 7:3 ratio. The average molecular weight was measured at Mw 140 000, Mn 36 900, and Mw/Mn 3.7 respectively, with the intrinsic viscosity of 1.3 dl/g. The degradation and resorption kinetics as well as the biocompatibility of injection molded devices made of poly (L-lactid-co-D, L-lactid) 70/30 has already been evaluated in several in vitro and in vivo studies. Experimental as well as clinical evaluation of the bioresorbable minipin was performed. Mass loss of the minipin was initiated after 6 months and it was completely metabolized by the body after 9 to 12 months without a clinically detectable foreign body reaction.

Keywords: guided bone regeneration, membrane fixation and stabilization, bioresorbable minipins

[1]Laboratory for Biomedical Engineering /Department of Orthopedic Surgery, National University of Singapore, 10 Kent Ridge Crescent, Singapore 119260
[2] Private Practice, Filderstadt, Talstr. 23, Germany
[3] Boehringer Ingelheim, Ingelheim am Rhein, Germany
[4] Department of Restorative Dentistry and Periodontology, Albert Ludwigs University, Freiburg, Hugstetterstr. 55, Germany

Introduction

Through the use of cell-occlusive membranes composed of non-resorbable materials, several authors [*1-4*] have introduced implant prosthetic treatment concepts in combination with Guided Bone Regeneration (GBR). Included among the most frequently-observed clinical complications are membrane collapse and wound dehiscence with an ensuing bacterial colonization of the membrane, which negatively influence the regeneration results [*5-7*].

Biomechanical stabilization and fixation of the membrane is a *conditio sine qua non* for wound healing in both soft and hard tissues. Nevins and Mellonig [*7*], as well as Wikesjö and Nilveus [*8*], have been able to demonstrate that micro-movements in the order of approximately 20 μm during the early healing phase prevent the differentiation of mesenchymal cells to osteoblasts, and thus cause these cells to become fibroblasts. Several authors have developed various membrane support and fixation systems, e.g., titanium mini-nails, mini-screws, titanium meshes and titanium plates, gold frames, and titanium-reinforced e-PTFE membranes [*2,7,9-12*]. The application of titanium mini-nails and mini-screws improves the membrane adaptation and limits the membrane's movement, while the meshes and the plate designs fundamentally support the space preservation under the membrane.

The disadvantage of the metallic and synthetic non-resorbable membranes and fixation systems is that a second operative maneuver is required to remove the material. Even with a minimally invasive procedure, the danger still exists that the newly regenerated hard tissue will be exposed and traumatized, thus provoking additional resorption [*13-15*]. To date, a series of membranes – manufactured from biomaterials composed of a natural or synthetic origin – have been investigated in both animal and clinical experiments [*16-23*]. In order to support and improve the biodegradable and bioresorbable membranes of their clinical efficacy, a bioresorbable minipin (Resor-Pin®, Geistlich, Wolhusen, Switzerland) and corresponding instruments have been developed to affix biodegradable and bioresorbable membranes (Figure 1a/b).

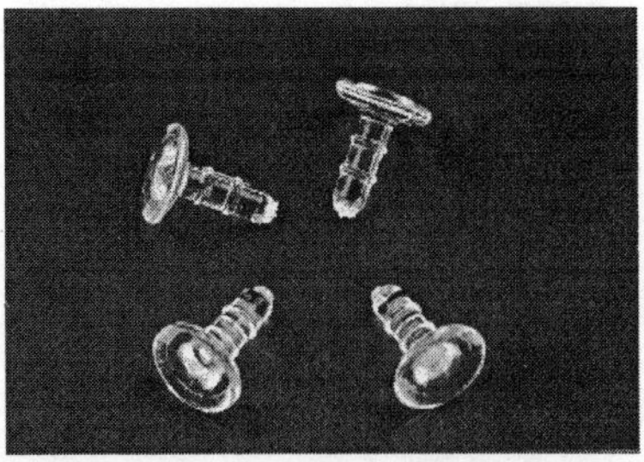

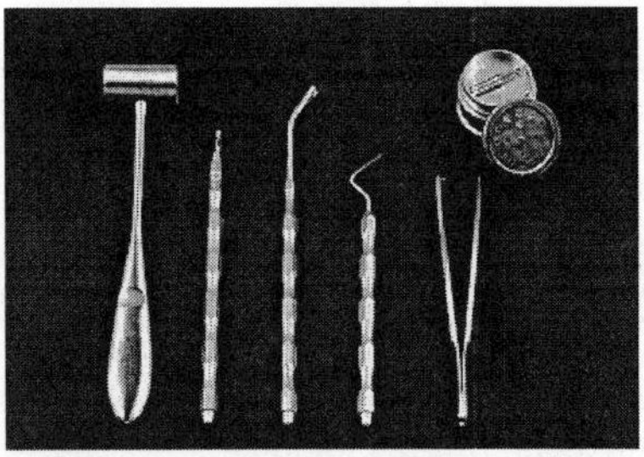

Figure 1a/b - *The bioresorbable minipin and the standard instrument set for inserting the bioresorbable minipin, consisting of hammer, membrane punch, membrane probe, straight and angled applicator, pin dispenser and drill.*

Biodegradation and Bioresorption

Within the past few years, aliphatic polyesters have prevailed as the largest group of synthetic bioresorbable polymers used in surgery. Those which should specifically be mentioned include polylactide, polyglcolide and polydiaxanone. Their number, diversity and large abundance of variation possibilities (copolymers, mixed polymers, softeners, additives, fiber reinforcements, etc.) also present a large advantage with regard to their usefulness as a membrane, and as a foil for guided tissue and guided bone regeneration. Hutmacher et al [*24*] reviewed those biodegradable and bioresorbable membranes that are currently commercially available for use in GTR and GBR techniques, as well as their material composition.

The terms biodegradable, bioresorbable, bioabsorbable and bioerodable are often used without a systematic classification or nomenclature in the literature that deals with guided tissue and bone regeneration. Vert [*25*] has provided a clear definition of these terms. The chronological course of the hydrolytic clearance process of aliphatic polyesters *in situ* can be described in five stages (Figure 2):

I. Hydration

The process of hydration initiated when the implant is inserted into the body. The gradient and the effect of the hydration are dependent on the chemical and physical structure of the biologically degradable implant. The mass and speed of the water uptake (diffusion) constitute the significant factors of the process. In the first phase, only those structures that are stabilized by van des Waal's forces and hydrogen bridges are attacked. As a side effect, one can observe how the water that has diffused in acts as a softener, e.g., the stability slightly decreases and the modulus of elasticity slightly increases. The primary foreign body reaction of biologically-degradable implants is determined by those same factors which govern non-degradable implants.

II. Hydration and Degradation (Loss of Stability)

The second phase of the degradation process is associated with an irreversible loss in toughness and stability of the implant. This commences as soon as the critical molecular weight is breached, which arises when the basic polymer structure is split into oligomers by the breakage of covalent bonds. The kinetics of both the loss in molecular weight and mass loss as well as the mechanical characteristics are likewise determined by the following factors: Chemical structure and composition, Presence of ionic groups and of side group defects, Configuration of the structure, Molecular weight and molecular weight distribution (polydispersity), Presence of low molecular weight components (monomers, oligomers, solvents, softeners, drugs, growth factors, etc.), Production and manufacturing procedures and their process parameters, Implant design, Sterilization method, Morphology (amorphous versus semi-crystalline, presence of microstructures and stress within the components), Tempering, Storage, Implant site.

III. Degradation (Loss of Shape and Mass)

In the third phase, the molecular weight decreases to the point that a fragmented and gelatin-like mass is formed, which displays no mechanical stability. Next, a splitting of the oligomers occurs, down to a molecular weight level, which cannot maintain the shape or the mass cohesion. At the end of this phase, the process which determines the secondary foreign body reaction begins, specifically, loss of mass.

IV. Resorption

In the fourth - and from a clinical standpoint, the most critical phase of the break-down process – the essential loss of implant mass occurs. Through a progressive hydrolysis, the gelatin-like particles are split into low molecular weight components. From a critical size downward, these can then be absorbed and assimilated by phagocytosis, and/or they become dissolved in the intracellular fluid.

V. Metabolization

In the final phase, a complete splitting of the compound into lactic acid and glycolic acid occurs, and these products then enter the citric acid cycle and are metabolized into carbon dioxide and pyruvate via an acetylation of co-enzyme A. The final metabolization of the molecules occurs via respiration and/or excretion of urine or solid waste.

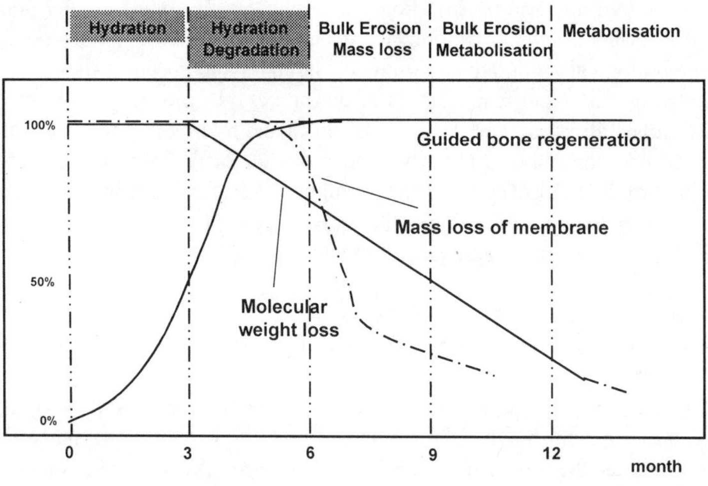

Figure 2 - *Graphic representation of the ideal degradation and resorption kinetics of membranes, minipins, etc., for hard tissue regeneration.*

Biodegradable and bioresorbable membranes for guided bone regeneration should maintain their physical barrier function for at least 6 months (Figure 2). From this, it follows that a similar requirement also applies to the degradation and resorption kinetics for a minipin used in the fixation of biodegradable or bioresorbable membranes. A number of research groups have investigated various polymers and copolymers composed of poly(L-lactide), poly(D, L-lactide) and polyglycolide with various molecular weights. These have been examined with respect to their degradation and resorption characteristics both *in vitro* and *in vivo* [*25-34*]. An evaluation of the data published in these studies revealed that the material, poly(L-lactide-co-D,L-lactide) 70/30, possesses the best-suited degradation and resorption kinetics for a minipin, which is to be used in membrane fixation.

An implant having the size and mass (5.4 mg) of the ResorPin loses its mechanical stability within a time frame of five to six months. It becomes completely metabolized by the body within 9 to 15 month, with a mass loss gradient (Figure 2) that do not initiate a clinically detectable secondary foreign body reaction. At 5 to 10 months after implantation, ResorPins (Figure 3a) and ResorPin heads (Figure 3b) were recovered in fourteen patients during secondary soft tissue surgery. The physical structure of the minipin was still completely intact after 5 to 6 month poly(L-lactide-co-D,L-lactide) 70/30. The milky coloring was a clear sign of an *in vivo* decrease in the molecular weight (Figure 3a). After 10 month in situ only degraded poly(L-lactide-co-D,L-lactide) 70/30 particles of the former minipin could be harvested. The determination of the molecular weight of the specimens, using Gel Permeation Chromatography (GPC), revealed the values listed in Table 1.

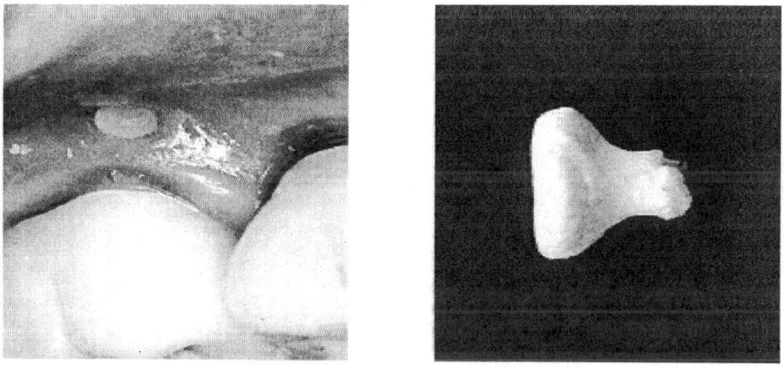

Figure 3 a/b - *Clinical situation of a mini-pin head seven months after implantation and the mini-pin head after drying and before determination of the molecular weight.*

Biocompatibility

Polylactides, polyglycolides and their copolymers are degraded and resorbed in the organism through non-specific hydrolysis to lactic acid and/or glycolic acid. Lactic acid is degraded in the citric acid cycle to carbon dioxide and water and then resorbed and metabolized. Glycolic acid is excreted with the urine or oxidized to glyoxylic acid under the influence of glycoloxidase. Glyoxylic acid is then converted through the intermediate

Table 1 - Data of the in situ molecular weight loss.

	time in situ	M_W	M_N	M_W/M_N
Poly (L-lactide-co-D,L-lactide) granule	-	1,082,100	440,800	2.4
Resor Pin before Gamma Sterilisation	-	420,600	191,700	2.2
Resor Pin after Gamma Sterilisation	-	384,400	166,200	2.4
Patient 1	10 month	36,700	13,500	2.72
Patient 2	6 month	135,200	35,900	3.77
Patient 3	6 month	139,200	36,900	3.8
Patient 4	8 month	55,400	26,800	2.1
Patient 5	8 month	52,200	25,400	2.1
Patient 6	8 month	53,400	23,600	2.3
Patient 7	8 month	60,200	27,600	2.2
Patient 8	11 month	9,400	4,700	2
Patient 9	10 month	37,700	13,300	2.8
Patient 10	8 month	57,000	19,300	2.9
Patient 11	6 month	137,000	36,500	3.8
Patient 12	7 month	94,000	32,500	2.9
Patient 13	6 month	132,800	36,100	3.7
Patient 14	7 month	92,400	30,900	3
Patient 15	7 month	93,100	31,700	2.9
Patient 15	10 month	27,000	8,800	3.1

stages, glycine and serine, into pyruvate as with lactic acid, can then be broken down in the citric acid cycle to carbon dioxide and water.

Investigations of tissue tolerability for bioresorbable polymers have been carried out in animal experiments using rats, mice, dogs and sheep. Suture materials made of bioresorbable polyesters have proven themselves in clinical application for more than 20 years. Retrospective, experience-based studies have pointed out the advantages with regard to low antigenicity, minimal tissue reaction, as well as the almost universal lack of formation of either abscesses or filamentous fistulae. Suture materials made from bioresorbable polyesters possess neither collagen-stimulating, antigenic nor pyrogenic characteristics. However, an increase in the cell populations of fibroblasts, histiocytes, lymphocytes and mast cells has been described in areas directly adjacent to the suture material. Occasionally, plasma cells and macrophages have also been reported. The mass loss of the material is accompanied by an increased migration of capillaries and phagocytizing cells, as well as an encapsulation of the thread material. This cell aggregation is reversible, i.e., cell accumulation decreases as the loss in mass of the polymer material progresses.

The material used for the minipin, poly(L-lactide-co-D,L-lactide) 70/30, has been examined in a large number of animal experiments and clinical studies [*24,26, 31,33-35*] All authors report that the copolymer is extremely biocompatible. Hürzeler *et al.* [*24,31*] used a bioresorbable minipin composed of poly(L-lactide-co-D,L-lactide) 70/30 in both animal and clinical experiments for the fixation of biodegradable collagen membranes and bioresorbable polyester membranes. After evaluation of the clinical and histological results, the authors concluded that, in these studies, the biologically degradable minipin demonstrated very good primary and secondary biocompatibility.

Minipin Design

Kirsch et al. [*9*] developed a metallic fixation system in order to support non-resorbable membranes with respect to a simplified clinical application, their space-preserving function, and tissue integration. The titanium membrane nail of the system, possessing a core diameter of 0.5 mm, has an ultraflat, lenticular head, and the retention groove with a diameter of 0.6 mm. The clinically-proven design concept of the titanium nail served as a template for the development of the biologically degradable minipin. Aliphatic polyesters have inferior mechanical characteristics in comparison to medical grade titanium[*9*]. Hence, the dimensions of the Resor-Pins were increased.

A polymer is in its most favorable form in the state of highest entropy when the individual molecular chains lie unordered in a ball-like structure. The macromolecules are present in an unordered form when the polymer mass is in its plastic state. During the shaping process, with the help of pressure and temperature (injection molding, extrusion, thermopressing, etc.), under the influence of shear and tensile forces, the macromolecules become primarily aligned in the direction of the flow of the melted mass. The injection of the polymer mass into a cooled mold enables an aligning and freezing of the polymer chains. In such a manner, the macromolecules are prevented from taking on the more favorable form of the ball-like structure. This phenomenon, which is strongly dependent on the polymer material and on the encompassing conditions, is described as orientation. The macromolecules possess the highest stability parallel to the orientation, whilst it is significantly decreased in the perpendicular direction.

The use of injection molding in the manufacturing of the bioresorbable minipins enabled the R&D team to consider the above-mentioned characteristics for a polymer material in the design concept. Biomedical engineers should implement the material-specific characteristics as well as the processing properties into their design concept when developing biologically resorbable devices and implants. The glass transition temperature of the material, poly(L-lactide-co-D,L-lactide), lies at between 45° to 55° C. Heating of the polymers towards their glass transition temperature leads to a relaxation of the polymer chains. These material characteristics further improve the (in addition to the retention ridges) stabilization of the Resor-Pins in the drill hole, and thus serves for an more applicable mechanical fixation and stabilization of the membranes.

Figure 4 shows two ResorPins on the injection cast, as they are ejected by the injection molding tool during manufacturing in the clean room. The injection molding tool was constructed in such a manner that the minipins were injected through the shaft apex, i.e., the direction of flow of the polymer glaze ran in an axial direction. The groove at the transition to the minipins has a diameter of 0.3 mm (compare with the ResorPin on the right side in Figure 4). If the injection molding parameters are set up in such a way that the tool was filled slowly, the minipin's molecular chains become highly oriented due to its small diameter.

Ideally, the polymer chains are arranged in a direction longitudinal to the pin shaft. *In situ,* the polymer implant undergoes a warming to body temperature within a short period of time. The relaxation of the polymer chains at a temperature of 37° C causes – via a shrinking in the radial direction - an expansion in the diameter of the shaft by 0.1 mm, and thus, to an additional bracing in the drill hole. In Figure 4, this behavior was simulated *in vitro* at a temperature of 70 ° C in order to facilitate visualization of the diameter expansion. From a manufacturing point of view, an additional advantage of the injection molding tool design is that the minipin no longer requires additional finishing after molding. Additional finishing processes would significantly increase the manufacturing costs as these also would have to take place under Clean Room conditions.

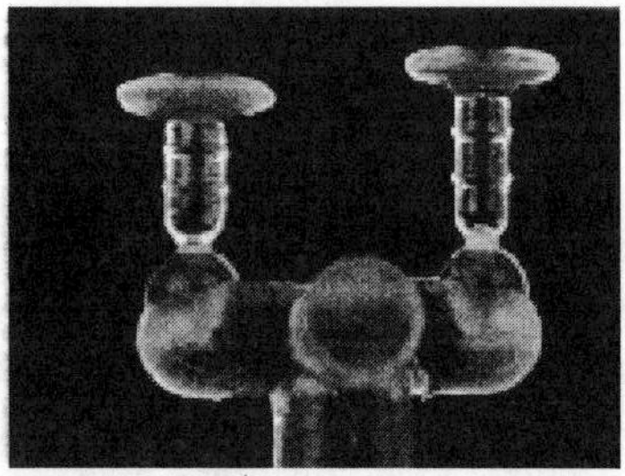

Figure 4 - *The ResorPin® as seen on the cast, after the injection processing. The relaxation of the polymer chains at a temperature of 37° C causes, via a shrinking/swelling process in the radial direction, an increase in the diameter of the ResorPin shaft by 0.1 mm. This then causes an additional bracing in the drill hole. This phenomenon is simulated in vitro at a temperature of 70° C in the two pins on the left, facilitating visualization of the shrinking/swelling principle.*

Mechanical Characteristics

The stability of bioresorbable polymers is significantly determined by the molecular weight, crystallinity, processing, thermal post-processing, sterilization, purity, remaining monomer content, moisture, surface structure and, with copolymers, the monomer composition. The stability values semi-crystalline polymers poly(L-lactide) and polyglycolide are significantly higher than the corresponding values of the low crystalline or amorphous polymers, poly-(D,L-lactide) and copolymers. The processing methods of extrusion, injection and compression molding, achieve the highest stability values. The decrease in stability values *in vitro* and *in vivo* is lower with the higher molecular polyesters than with those having lower molecular weights. With inherent viscosities above 1.0 dl/g, it is primarily the above-mentioned factors that determine the reduction in the mechanical properties.

A study carried out by Claes *et al.* [*26*] revealed the following data: after injection molding and after sterilization with gamma radiation, the material chosen for the bioresorbable minipin, poly(L-lactide-co-D, L-lactide) 70/30, showed a MW of 164 000 and 187 000 as well as a bending strength of 155 to 163 MPa, respectively. An average molecular weight of MW 140 000 and an average inherent viscosity of 1.3 dl/g were measured for the ResorPin using different batches after injection molding and sterilization with gamma radiation.

Clinical data

Between January 1, 1996 and July 31, 1999, some 657 bioresorbable minipins were inserted for the fixation and stabilization of 148 double-layer collagen membranes in 106 patients of a German private practice. On average, 4.9 minipins were inserted per patient, whereby the minimum was 2 and the maximum was 19. In none of the patients a clinically-detectable primary or secondary foreign body reaction was noticeable.

The indications for implementing guided bone regeneration into the implant prosthetic treatment concept were divided into the following: monocortical block removal from chin 23, monocortical block removal from the retromolar area: 3, augmentation after sinus floor elevation 41, augmentation of the alveolar process with monocortical blocks: 27, dehiscence after implant placement: 53.

The average age of the 106 patients was 50.9 years, the youngest being 19-years-old and the oldest, 78-years-old. Some 50.9% (54) of the patients were women with an average age of 49.1 years and 49,1% (52) men with an average age of 52.9 years. Today, approximately 75.000 ResorPins, which have been approved according to FDA and European standards (CS Mark), have been inserted in a clinical setting. Based on both literature survey and from correspondences with clinicians, the authors know of no case where there has been a clinically detectable foreign body reaction due to the bioresorbable minipin. On account of the mechanical properties it is important that the minipin is inserted parallel to the axis of the drilled hole. Otherwise pin breakage during insertion may occur.

The following clinical cases (Figure 5-9) demonstrate the implementation of the process of guided bone regeneration while using biodegradable biomaterials in surgically-challenging implant prosthetic treatment regimes.

Case 1

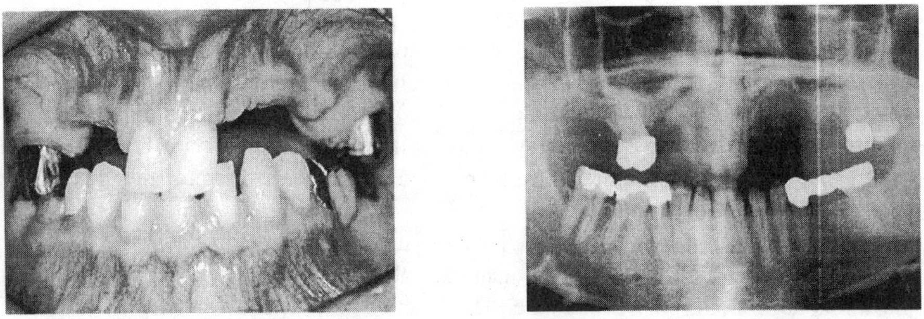

Figure 5 a/b - *A 27-year-old female patient presented with a genuine hypodontia. Due to the lack of teeth, the alveolar process was incompletely developed. The unfavorable intermaxillary relationships are clearly evident in the orthopantomogram (Figure 5b). As the large gaps present bilaterally demonstrated inadequate volume for the alveolar processes, an implant prosthetic provision was not possible without first undergoing augmentation of the alveolar process via guided bone regeneration. The orthopantomogram emphasizes the unfavorable inter-maxillary relationships. The occlusal view shows the asymmetrical course of the alveolar process in the partially-edentulous maxilla. The oro-vestibular bone deficit could only be compensated by using autologous bones grafts.*

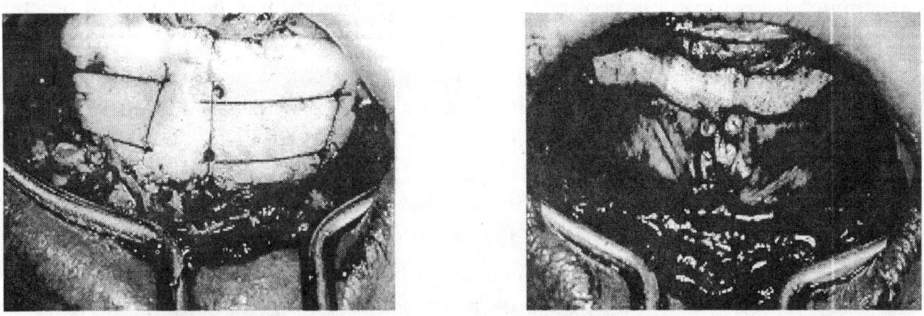

Figure 6 a/b - *After a multi-layered soft tissue preparation at the chin underneath the root apices of the mandibular front teeth, two corticospongious block transplants were removed. After the graft removal, the defect was initially filled with an augmentation material and secondarily covered with a biodegradable collagen membrane, which was fixed with bioresorbable pins.*

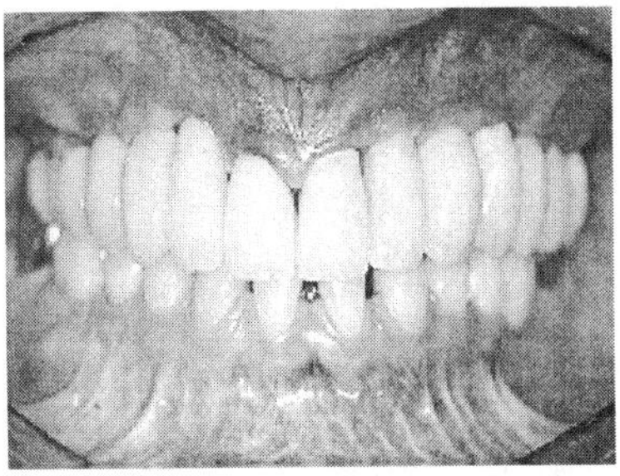

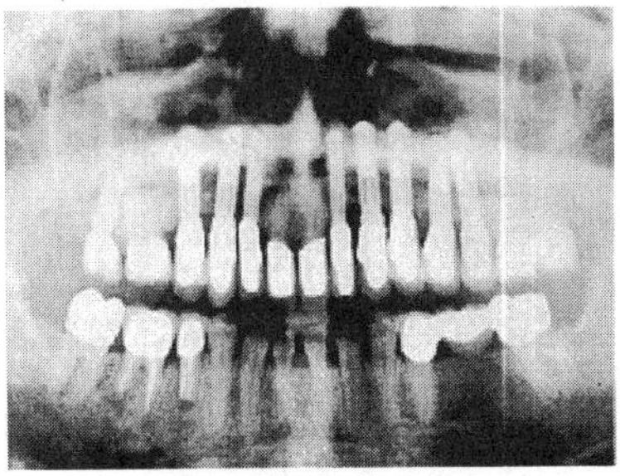

Figure 7a/b - *In the occlusal view, one can recognize the individually manufactured aesthetic superstructures and the inflammation-free peri-implant soft tissue relationships. In comparison to the initial situation, the already almost symmetrically-shaped dental arch can be seen here. As part of the definitive restoration, the metal-ceramic individual tooth crowns were attached using cement on the aesthetic superstructures. The orthopantomogram taken immediately after inserting the definitive restoration emphasizes the clinical success of the guided bone regeneration treatment.*

Case 2

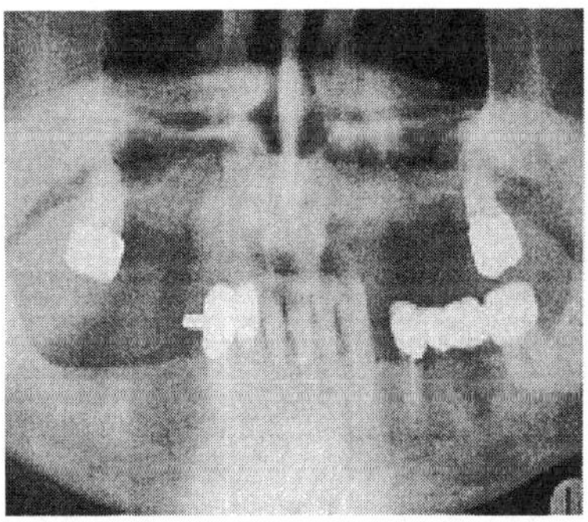

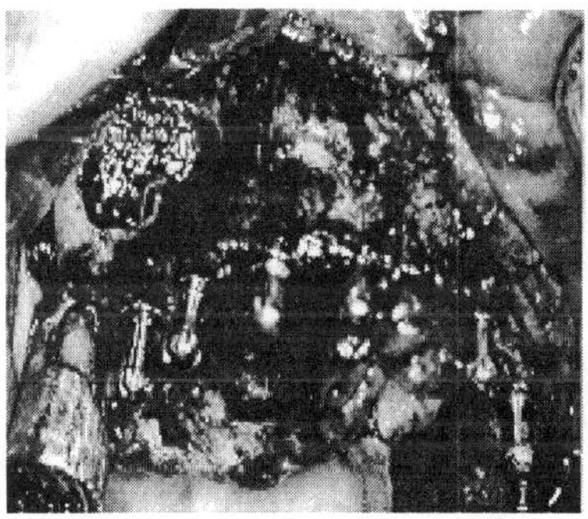

Figure 8a/b - *In January 1997, a 65-year-old patient presented with periodontal, dental and occlusal problems. Even though the patient made a youthful impression, a multitude of pathological processes, already ongoing for several years, had ultimately led to a situation in which the original function of stomatognathic system could no longer be carried out. The orthopantomogram highlights the clinical findings (Figure 8a). After the placement of implants in the area of the maxillary front teeth, buccal fenestrations appeared which were covered with a xenogenous bone substitution material (Figure 8b).*

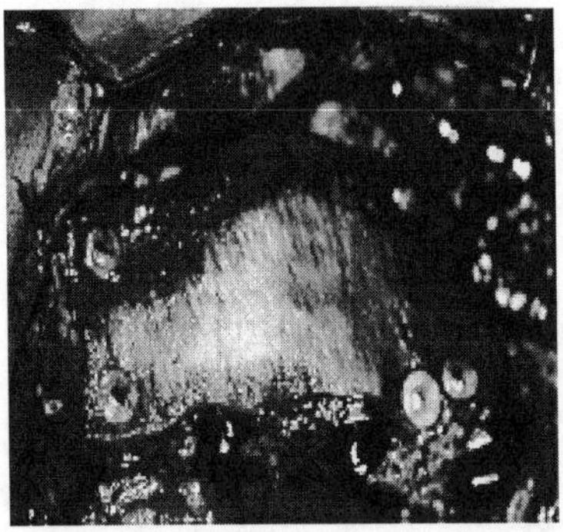

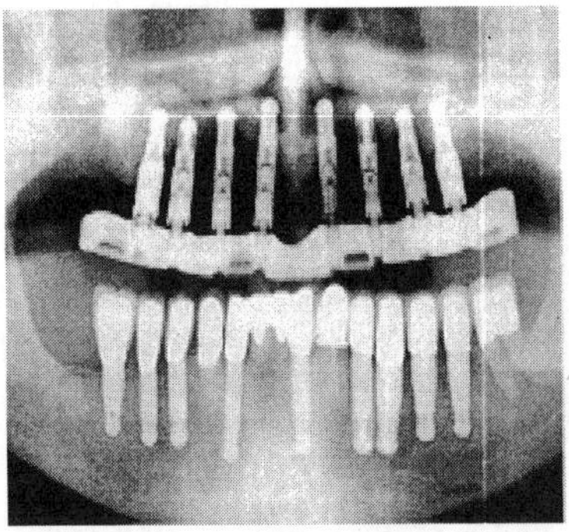

Figure 9a/b - *Subsequently, a double-layer collagen membrane was inserted. This served for securing the positioning and for promoting bony healing of the xenogenous augmentation material as part of the guided bone regeneration. For stabilization purposes, the collagen membrane was stabilized with five Resor-Pins (Figure 9a). The membrane probe simplifies insertion of the minipins. The insertion of an adequate number of bioresorbable minipins – in general, four to six minipins per membrane – prevents a relative movement between the membrane and the surrounding bone and/or between the membrane and the mucoperiosteal flaps. The orthopantomogram taken eight months after implantation highlights the clinical success of the total rehabilitation process (Figure 9b).*

Discussion

During the past three years, comprehensive reports dealing with the clinical application of biodegradable and bioresorbable membranes in GTR and GBR techniques have been documented in literature [*31-37*]. Hutmacher et al [*38*] reviewed the GTR/GBR membranes that are currently commercially available, their experimental and clinical data as well as their material composition. A large majority of the membranes were originally developed for use in guided tissue regeneration (GTR). The requirements posed for the degradation and resorption kinetics [*38,39,40*], occlusivity and space preservation, which are demanded of biodegradable and bioresorbable membranes for guided bone regeneration differ from those of membranes used in guided tissue regeneration.

The degradation and resorption kinetics for a membrane which is to be used for guided bone regeneration should be tailored in such a manner that it remains intact for at least six months - and with large volume bony defects, for nine months – and then it should become completely metabolized after 12 to 15 months [*40*]. With the exception of a double-layer collagen membrane, none of the commercially available membranes fulfills this requirement. A great number of membranes have been originally developed for GTR where a physical barrier function of 4 to 6 weeks is adequate [*38*]. The fixation and stabilization of biodegradable and bioresorbable membranes is only practical when used in combination with bioresorbable fixation devices. Otherwise, the advantages offered – such as avoiding a second operation or the minimally invasive procedure of inserting endosseal implants – are made redundant.

In a clinical study, Lundgren *et al.* [*20*] examined a bioresorbable membrane designed for the GTR technique in combination with implants for the GBR technique. A foil composed of polyhydroxybutyrate was tested in rat models, specifically investigating their suitability for the regeneration of mandibular defects [*23, 36*]. Polyhydroxybutyrate is mainly broken down through an enzymatic hydrolysis. Therefore, these polymers possess degradation and metabolization kinetics lasting between several years to decades [*30*], and are thus not appropriate for use as implant materials. Using a rat model, Sandberg *et al.* [*21*] examined membranes that had the same design, but three different copolymer compositions based on polyglycolide and poly-(L-lactide) in "critical size defects". The membrane with the highest poly(L-lactide) proportion showed degradation and resorption kinetics which were suitable for guided bone regeneration. However, the authors provided no precise information regarding the material composition, molecular weight, design, etc.

One currently available biodegradable membrane for use in the GBR technique composed of highly purified porcine collagen types I and III, was examined by different teams with the application of bioresorbable minipins using both animal experiments and clinical studies [*3,24,38,39*]. All membrane types described above required an osteoconductive and/or osteoinductive filling material for building up the peri-implant defects and for preventing membrane collapse. The precise membrane adaptation to the surrounding bone is critical in order that the soft tissue cells of the covering mucosa do not gain access to the bone defects. This ensures that the regeneration of the newly-formed bone is not hampered. Adaptation to the surrounding bone surface is significantly facilitated through the stabilization of the biodegradable or bioresorbable membrane with minipins composed of poly(L-lactide-co-D,L-lactide) 70/30. With the application of membranes/foils which become more flexible *in situ*, one end of the membrane can be fixed with a bioresorbable minipin, then stretched over the bone defect, such as in the form of a tent or a hood. This enables the oral surgeon to achieve a tight closure and a wrinkle-free appositional transition of the physical barrier device to the host bone and/or periosteum. In this way, one ensures that no micro-movements of the membrane occurs – neither on the bone side nor on the soft tissue side - which is a *conditio sine qua non* for successful GBR treatment regime.

Conclusions

Over the past ten years extensive experimental and clinical testing has been performed on devices and implants made of poly(L-lactide-co-D,L-lactide) 70/30. The aliphatic copolymer material has been found to be non-toxic, non-mutagenic, non-irritating, and non-pyrogenic. The clinical results of this non-randomized study demonstrate that the ResorPin provides adequate material and design properties to be used as a membrane fixation device.

References

[1] Mellonig J.T., Nevins M., Guided bone regeneration of bone defects associated with implants: An evidence-based outcome assessment. J Periodontics Restorative Dentistry 1995; Vol.15:169-184.

[2] Buser D., Dula, K., Hirt, H.P., Berthold, H., "Localized ridge augmentation using guided bone regeneration", Buser, D., Dahlin, C., Schenk, K.R. (eds.), Guided bone regeneration in implant dentistry, Quintessence, 1994, pp 189-234.

[3] Jovanovic S.A, Buser D. "Guided bone regeneration in dehiscence defects and delayed extraction sockets", Buser, D., Dahlin, C., Schenk, K.R. (eds.), Guided bone regeneration in implant dentistry, Quintessence, 1994, pp 189-234.

[4] Schenk R.K, Buser D, Hardwick WR, Dahlin C. Healing pattern of bone regeneration in membrane protected defects. Int J Oral Maxillofac Implants 1994; 9:13-29.

[5] Weingart D, Schilli W., Operative Techniken zur Verhinderung des Membrankolapses bei der gesteuerten Knochenregneration., Implantologie 1994; 3: 223-23.

[6] Simion M., Trisi P., Piatelli A, Vertical ridge augmentation using a membrane technique associated with osseointegrated implants. Int J Periodont Restorative Dent 1994; 4:497-511.

[7] Nevins M., Mellonig J., Enhancement of the damaged edentoulus ridge to receive dental implants: A combination of allograft and the Gore-tex membrane. Int. J Periodont Rest Dent 1992; 12:97-111.

[8] Wikesjö U., Nilveus R., Periodontal repair in dogs: Effect of wound stabilization on healing. J Periodontol 1990; 61:719-724.

[9] Kirsch A., Ackermann K. L., Hürzeler M. B., Dürr W., Hutmacher D., Gesteuerte Knochenregeneration - 5 Jahre klinische Erfahrung mit der Applikation von Titanmembrannägeln zur Fixation von nicht-resorbierbaren Membranen. Implantologie 1996; 4: 289-297.

[10] Tinti C., Parma-Benfenati S., Manfrini F., Metallstrukturen als Platzhalter für nicht resorbierbare Membranen bei gesteuerter Knochenregeneration um Implantate. Zwei Fallschilderungen. Int J Periodont Restorative Dent 1997; 17:53-61.

[11] von Arx T., Hardt N., Wallkamm K. B., Die Time-Technik: Lokale Osteoplastik zur Alveolarkammaugmentation – Auswertung und Ergebnisse der ersten 15 Fälle. Implantologie 1996; 1:33-48.

[12] Meltzer A.M, Edenbaum D.R.,Alveolarkammaugmentation gestützt mit dreidimensionalen Mikroplatten – eine Alternative zur Nervtransposition. Parodontol Rest Zahnheilkd 1997; 17:257-265.

[13] Ramfjord, S., Costich, E.: Healing after exposure of periosteum on the alveolar process. J Periodontol 39, 199-203, 1968.

[14] Melcher, A.H., Accursi, G.E.: Osteogenic capacity of periosteal and osteoperiosteal flaps elevated from the parietal bone of the rat. Arch Oral Biol 16, 573-574, 1971.

[15] Carranza, F.A. Jr., Carraro, J.J.: Effects of removal of periosteum on postoperative results in mucogingival surgery. J Periodontol 34, 223-229, 1963.

[16] Lundgren D., Laurell L., Gottlow J., Rylander H., Mathisen H., Nyman S., Rask M.: The influence of the design of two different bioresorbable barriers on the results of guided tissue regeneration therapy. An intra-individual comparative study in the monkey. J Peridontol 1995; 66:605-612
[17] Warrer K., Guided tissue regeneration in recession type defects using a bioabsorbable RESOLUT or non-bioabsorbable GORE-TEX Periodontal material (GTPM) membranes. J Dental Research 1994; 73 (special issue):380.
[18] Gottlow J., Guided tissue regeneration using bioresorbable and non-resorbable devices: Initial healing and long-term results. J Peridontol 1993; 64:1157-1165.
[19] Polson A.M., Southard G.L., Dunn R.D., Polson A.P., Billen J.R., Laster L.L., Initial study of guided tissue regeneration in Class II furcation defects after use of a biodegradable barrier. Int J Periodont Rest Dentistry 1995; 15:43-55.
[20] Lundgren D., Sennerby L, Falk H, Friberg B, Nyman S: The use of a new bioresorbable barrier for guided bone regeneration in connection with implant installation. Clin Oral Im Res 1994; 3:177-184.
[21] Sandberg E., Dahlin C., Linde A., Bone regeneration by the ostepromotion technique using bioabsorbable membranes: An experimental study in rats. J Oral Maxillofac Surg 1993; 51:1106-1114.
[22] Gotfredsen K., Nimb L., Hjorting-Hansen E., Immediate implant placement using a biodegradable barrier, polyhydroxybutyrate-hydroxyvalerate reinforced with Polyglactin 910. Clin Oral Imp Res 1994; 5:83-91.
[23] Hürzeler M.B., Weng D., Hutmacher D. Knochenregeneration um Implantate – eine klinische Studie mit einer neuen resorbierbaren Membran. Dtsch Zahnärztl Z 1996; 51:298-303.
[24] Hutmacher D., Huerzeler M.B., Schliephake H., A Review of Material Properties of Biodegradable and Bioresorbable Polymers and Devices for GTR and GBR Applications. Int J Oral Maxillofac Implants 1996, Vol 11:667-678
[25] Vert M., Bioresorbable polymers for temporary therapeutic applications. Angew Makrom Ch 1989, Vol 167:155-168.
[26] Claes L., Ignatius A.A., Rehm K.E., Scholz C.,A new biodegradable pin for the reduction of bony fragments: design, mechanical properties and in vitro degradation. Biomaterials 1996, Vol 17 No. 16, pp 1621-1626
[27] Gutwald R., Pistner H., Reuther J., Muehling J., Biodegradation and tissue reaction in long term implantation study of poly (L-lactide). J Mat Scie Med 1994, 5:485-490.
[28] Varlet-Mainil P., Cordey J., Gogolewski S., Positional stability of polylactidee pins with various surface textures in sheep tibia. J Biomedical Mat Research, 1997, Vol 34:351-359.
[29] Bergsma J.E., Rozema F.R., Bos R.R.M., Boering G., Bruijn W, C., Late degradation tissue response to poly (L-lactide) bone plates and screws. Biomaterials 1995, Vol. 16:25-31.
[30] Holland S.J., Tighe B.J., Gould P.L., Polymers for biodegradable medical devices, I. The potential of polyesters as controlled macromolecular release systems. J Control Rel 1986, Vol 4:155-163.

[31] Hürzeler M.B., Strub J.R., Guided bone regeneration around exposed implants: a new bioresorbable device and bioresorbable membrane pins. Practical Periodontics Aesth Dentistry 1995; 7(10):37-47.

[32] Bostman O., Hirvensalo E., Makinen J., Rokkanen P., Foreign body reaction to fracture fixation implants of biodegradable synthetic polymers. J Bone Joint Surg (Br) 1990; 72-B:592.

[33] Schliephake H., Neukam W.F, Hutmacher D., Becker J., Enhancement of bone ingrowth into a porous hydroxyapatite-matrix using a resorbable polylactic membrane. J Oral Maxillofac Surg 1994; 52:57-63.

[34] Schliephake H, Neukam W F, Hutmacher D, Whstenfeld H: Experimental transplantation of HA-bone composite grafts. J Oral Maxillofac Surg 1994; 53:46-51

[35] Schliephake H., Neukam W. F., Hutmacher D., Becker J., The use of a basic fibroblast growth factor (bFGF) for enhancement of bone ingrowth into pyrolized bovine bone. Int J Oral Maxillofac Surg 1994; 52:57-63

[36] Kostopoulos L., Karring T., Augmentation of the rat mandible using guided tissue regeneration. Clin Oral Impl Res 1994: 5:75-82.

[37] Zitzmann N.U., Naef R., Schärer P., Resorbable Membranes in Combination with BioOss for Guided Bone Regeneration. Int J Oral Maxillofac Implants 1997; 12:844-852.

[38] Hürzeler M.B., Kohal, R.J., Naghshbandi, J., Mota, L.F., Conradt, J., Hutmacher, D., Caffesse, R.G. Evaluation of a new bioresorbable barrier to fascilitate bone regeneration around exposed implant threads. An experimental study in the monkey. Int J Oral Maxillofac Surg 1998; 27: 315-320.

[39] Hutmacher D.W., Kirsch A., Ackermann, K.L., Huerzeler M.B., A Tissue Engineered Cell Occlusive Device for Hard Tissue Regeneration – A Preliminary Report. Int J Periodontics Restorative Dent (in press)

C. Mauli Agrawal,[1] James S. McKinney,[1] Dingyi Huang,[1] and Kyriacos A. Athanasiou[1]

The Use of the Vibrating Particle Technique to Fabricate Highly Porous and Permeable Biodegradable Scaffolds

---

Reference: Agrawal, C. M., McKinney, J. S., Huang, D., and Athanasiou, K. A., **"The Use of the Vibrating Particle Technique to Fabricate Highly Porous and Permeable Biodegradable Scaffolds,"** *Synthetic Bioabsorbable Polymers for Implants, ASTM STP 1396,* C. M. Agrawal, J. E. Parr, and S. T. Lin, Eds., American Society for Testing and Materials, West Conshohocken, PA, 2000.

Abstract: This study describes the degradation behavior of biodegradable scaffolds fabricated from a copolymer of polylactic acid and polyglycolic acid using a new technique that eliminates some of the problematic issues with the salt-leaching technique. Two variations of this technique were used and the *in vitro* degradation characteristics of the resulting scaffolds were compared. The properties monitored included mass, molecular weight, porosity, permeability, mechanical stiffness, and polydispersity. The results indicated that the vibrating particle technique, results in scaffolds that are at least 90% porous and highly permeable. During degradation the porosity of the scaffolds initially decreased up to two weeks and then inceased. On the other hand, their stiffness first increased followed by a decrease. It was also determined that the permeability of the scaffolds can vary considerably without significant changes in the porosity.

Keywords: degradation, scaffold, tissue engineering, polylactic acid, biodegradable

Introduction

One of the strategies currently used in tissue engineering orthopaedic tissues is to provide musculoskeletal cells with a biodegradable scaffold or framework for attachment, proliferation and ultimately extracellular matrix formation. It is generally

---

[1]Associate Professor of Orthopaedics & Engineering, research student, research assistant, and Associate Professor of Orthopaedics & Engineering, respectively, Department of Orthopaedics-7774, The University of Texas Health Science Center at San Antonio, 7703 Floyd Curl Drive, San Antonio, Texas 78229-3900

accepted that the ideal scaffold should be biocompatible, resorbable, and highly porous (>90%). Furthermore, it should maintain its three-dimensional structure during resorption, have a predetermined degradation rate, and should facilitate cell adhesion and growth [*1*]. The architecture or morphological properties of the scaffold are critical to ensuring its efficacy in tissue engineering applications. Among others, the porosity and permeability of the scaffold play important roles in its success. A highly porous structure provides the pathways for cellular infiltration and space for extracellular matrix formation. On the other hand, high scaffold permeability facilitates inward diffusion of nutrients, as well as the removal of degradation products and metabolic waste. Freed et al. [*2*] determined that high porosity was better suited for cartilage regeneration. However, during the design process, changing the porosity of a biodegradable scaffold may significantly alter other properties, such as its permeability and degradation kinetics [*3*]. Changing scaffold permeability may also result in similar outcomes. Thus, both porosity and permeability are important aspects of scaffold design and are determined, to a large extent, by the technique used for fabricating the scaffold.

Numerous scaffold fabrication techniques have been described in the literature and several use biodegradable polylactic acid (PLA) and polyglycolic acid (PGA) materials [*4*]. Mikos et al. [*5*] have described a salt-leaching technique that involves adding a water soluble porogen, such as NaCl crystals, to a PLA-PGA polymer solution in a mold. The solution is then evaporated and the polymer-salt solid is immersed in water to remove the salt. This popular technique is relatively easy to implement and yields specimens with good overall porosity. However, in our hands, this technique usually results in non-uniform porosity unless the scaffold is very thin. Also, in our experience, scaffolds fabricated using this technique usually have a thin polymeric film on one end which occludes the pores.

The objective of the present study was to characterize PLA-PGA scaffolds fabricated using the novel vibrating particle technique, which eliminates some of the issues, described above, related to the salt-leaching technique. As a first step in the characterization of these scaffolds, their physical and mechanical properties, and *in vitro* degradation behavior were examined and are reported here.

Materials and Methods

Implant Production

Two groups of 5 mm (diameter) x 3 mm (height) PLA-PGA disk-shaped scaffolds were fabricated employing a new technique, which uses vibrating particles to enhance porosity and permeability. Two different particle-to-polymer ratios (w/w) were used to assess their effect on the morphology and degradation of the resulting scaffolds. Also, one set of six scaffolds were fabricated using the standard salt-leaching technique without the vibrating particles. These six were used for initial comparison only and were not subjected to degradation tests.

To make the first group of implants (Group A), 0.125 gm of 50/50 poly(DL-lactide-co-glycolide) (Birmingham Polymers Inc., Birmingham, AL. Lot# D96026) with an inherent viscosity of 0.70 dl/gm and weight average molecular weight of 62 kDa was dissolved in 3 mL of pure acetone under continuous stirring. Next, 2.0 gm of sodium chloride (NaCl) particles (250 μm ≤ salt size ≤ 500 μm) were spread evenly at the bottom of a Teflon mold with a rectangular cavity or well (33 x 20 x 15 mm). The polymer (PLG) solution was then poured evenly onto the salt in the well; the mold was next placed under continuous air flow conditions and vibrated using a Thermolyne Maxi Mix II (Barnstead/Thermolyne. Dubuque, IA) for 7 minutes. At this point, another 2.0 gm of NaCl were evenly added to the mold, which was gently vibrated for an additional 3 minutes. Finally, 1.0 gm of salt was evenly introduced over the now semi-solid polymer in the well. The open mold was left standing for an additional hour and then placed in a heated vacuum at 45°C and 5000 mTorr for 24 hours. After the 24 hour period, cylindrical scaffolds were extracted from the solid polymer-salt composite in the mold with a 5 mm diameter punch and placed in distilled water (replaced every 12 hours) for 72 hours, to dissolve the NaCl. After removal from the water, the implants were dried in a vacuum and stored at –20°C until testing. The salt to polymer ratio for Group A scaffolds was approximately 40:1.

For Group B scaffolds, the salt to polymer ratio was 14:1, which was approximately three times less than for Group A. In this case, 0.77 gm of the same PLG polymer described above was dissolved in 6.5 mL of acetone. The polymer solution was then poured over 4.5 gm of salt in the Teflon mold, which was vibrated for a total of 8.5 minutes under constant air flow conditions. During this period, an additional 4.5 g of salt were added after 3.75 minutes of shaking, and 2.0 gm at 7.0 minutes. The mold was left under controlled air flow for 24 hours and then placed in a heated vacuum at 45°C and 5000 mTorr for 24 hours. The scaffolds were extracted using a 5 mm punch, immersed in water for 48 hours, and then dried in a vacuum.

A separate set of six implants were fabricated using exactly the same procedure described above for Group B, but without vibrating the particles. These were designated as Group C.

Degradation

For Groups A and B, 56 scaffolds each were fabricated. Furthermore, each group was subdivided into 7 subgroups of 8 specimens each, corresponding to degradation times of 0, 1, 2, 3, 4, 6 and 8 weeks. Each scaffold was weighed and placed in an individual 15 mL glass centrifuge tube containing 10 mL of phosphate buffered saline, pH 7.4, at 37°C. Every 3.5 days, the PBS was changed to avoid the build-up of degradation products and accompanying changes in pH. At the end of each test period, a set of implants from both Groups A and B was removed from the PBS, dried in a vacuum, and analyzed as described below.

Mass

The mass of the implants was measured on an electronic balance with a resolution of 1 μg.

Permeability

Permeability was measured using a direct permeation experiment which measures the rate of flow of water through the implant under a known hydrostatic pressure head. This information, in conjunction with Darcy's Law, was used to calculate the permeability as described earlier [*6*].

Porosity

Porosity of the scaffolds was measured using the Archimedes' Principle. After determining its dry mass, the scaffold was pre-wet by placing it in ethanol under negative pressure. It was then saturated with water using the same procedure; the implant was then removed from the water and weighed to determine its wet mass. Next it was completely immersed in water and its submerged mass was measured. Percent porosity was then calculated as follows.

$$\%\text{Porosity} = (M_{wet} - M_{dry})/(M_{wet} - M_{submerged})$$

Molecular Weight

Changes in the weight average molecular weight of the polymer were determined as a function of degradation time using gel permeation chromatography (GPC). Cross sections of the scaffolds, approximately 3 mg in weight, were dissolved in 1 mL of chloroform, filtered using a micropore filter (0.45 μm) and analyzed using GPC. The system used chloroform as the mobile phase and polystyrene standards.

Polydispersity

At each degradation time point the polydispersity of the polymer was measured by gel permeation chromatography, using the technique described above.

Mechanical Properties

The stiffness of the implants was tested by creep indentation using an automated stress-relaxation creep indentation (ASCI) apparatus developed in our laboratory [*7*]. The PLG implants were pre-wet as described earlier, placed in a sample holder, and immersed in deionized water. After the application of a 9.81×10^{-3} N tare load, a 29.4×10^{-3} N perpendicular, compressive, step load was applied through a 1.5 mm diameter porous, rigid, indenter tip. The maximum displacement, indenter tip radius, load applied, and specimen thickness were used as variables in the Boussinesq-Papkovitch equation, which was used to calculate the elastic modulus of the specimen

$$E = P(1 - v^2)/2aw_o$$

where E is the Young's modulus (MPa), P is the load applied (N), ν is the Poisson's ratio (assumed to be 0.3 for this study), a is the radius of the loading tip (mm), and w_o is the maximum creep deformation.

Size and Morphology

The size of the scaffolds was determined by measuring their diameter and height using calipers. Micrographs of the implants were taken by a scanning electron microscope to study temporal microscopic structural changes of both the interior and exterior of the implants as they degrade over time. To accomplish this task, the specimens were frozen in liquid nitrogen for 60 seconds and then cut in a guillotine-like apparatus to obtain a cross-section. These samples were then sputter coated with gold-palladium and imaged in a Philips (JEOL Inc. Peabody, MA) 500 scanning electron microscope at 15 kV. The highly porous nature of Group B scaffolds before degradation is shown in Fig. 1.

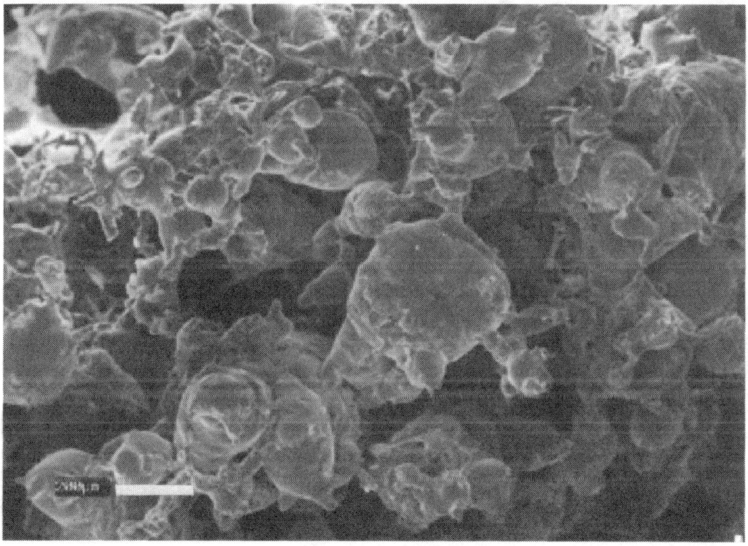

Fig. 1 – *Scanning electron micrograph of Group B Scaffold prior to degradation showing porosity and interconnected pores. White bar denotes 100μm.*

Statistical Analysis

All data were arranged as mean ± standard deviation. Significant differences were determined using analysis of variance (ANOVA) and Fisher's least significant difference test as needed.

Results

Comparison of Groups B and C

Specimens from Group B (vibrating-particle method) and Group C (salt-leaching technique) were compared for their morphology, porosity, and permeability. Group C specimens had a thin film occluding the pores on one side as shown in Fig. 2. Group B specimens, on the other hand, had no film and had clear, open pores on either end of the specimen (Fig. 3). Moreover, unlike the Group B specimens, Group C specimens demonstrated a definite change in pore morphology from one end to the other when longitudinal cuts of the scaffolds were examined. This gradient may be due to the gravity-assisted settling of salt particles during solvent evaporation in Group C.

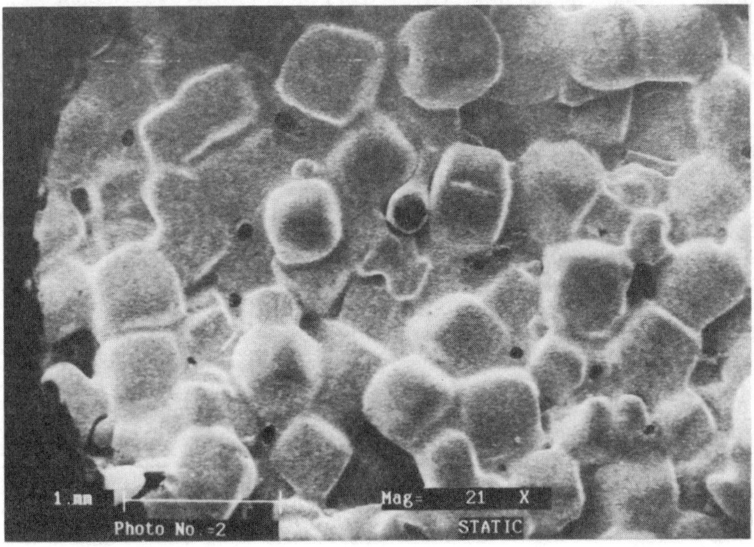

Fig. 2 – *Group C specimens were fabricated using the standard salt-leaching technique and exhibited a film occluding one side. This film significantly decreased the permeability of the specimens.*

Table 1 shows a comparison of the porosity and permeability values for Groups B and C. It is clear that although the porosity for the two types of scaffolds is comparable, their permeability values are vastly different. This may be due to the existence of the polymeric film on one end of Group C specimens (salt-leaching).

Comparison of Groups A and B

Changes in the permeability of scaffolds as a function of degradation time are shown in Fig. 4. The permeability of Groups A and B at t = 0 was 2.39±1.49 (E-08 $m^4/N{\cdot}s$) and 24.4±11.3 (E-08 $m^4/N{\cdot}s$), respectively, which indicated a ten-fold

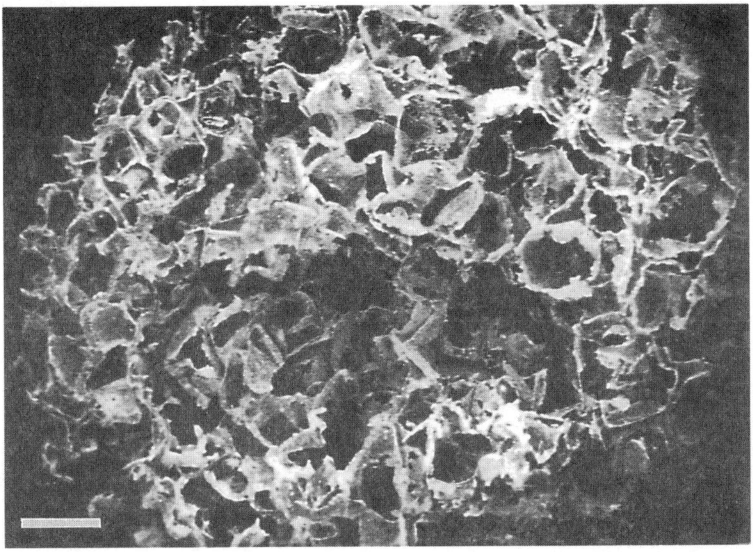

Fig. 3 – *Group B specimens were fabricated using the new vibrating-particle technique which eliminates non-porous films and results in uniform porosity throughout the thickness of the specimen. White bar denotes 500μm.*

difference. At Week 4, Group A specimens were too soft and friable to perform permeability tests. Group B specimens reached the same state, but only after six weeks of degradation.

Table 1-*Comparison of vibrating-particle and salt-leaching techniques.*

Scaffold Type	Porosity	Permeability (E-08 $m^4/N{\cdot}s$)
Group B (vibrating-particle)	91.8 ± 1.6	24.4 ± 11.3
Group C (salt-leaching)	92.9 ± 1.1	1.91 ± 0.84

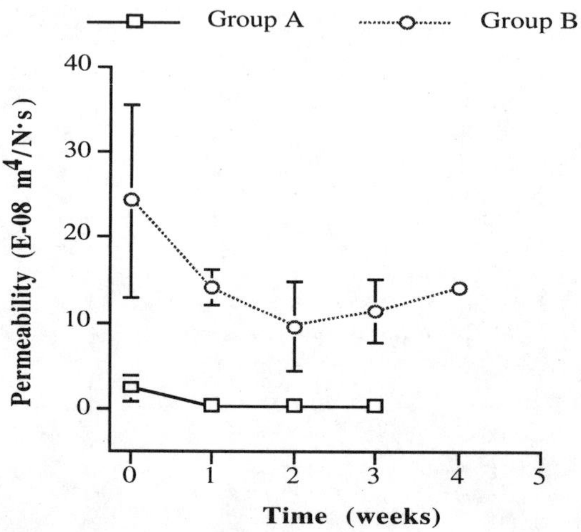

Fig. 4 - *Changes in the permeability of the scaffolds as function of degradation time. Scaffolds in Group B were significantly more permeable compared to Group A.*

The changes in porosity as a function of time are shown in Fig. 5. At t = 0 Group A scaffolds comprised a highly interconnected, highly porous system with a porosity of 93.1±0.7%. The porosity decreased up to Week 2 for this group and then started to increase again. Specifically, the porosity decreased to 87.2±1.4% at Week 1 and 77.7±3.9% at Week 2. At Week 3 there was an increase to 90.6±2.7%. By Week 4, the implants were too fragile to undergo testing. Group B specimens demonstrated a similar pattern of change in porosity through Week 3. However, this group maintained sufficient mechanical strength to enable testing up to Week 6. The porosity increased to 95.2±1.3% at Week 4 and then decreased again to 85.5±3.7% by Week 6.

Mass

There was no significant mass loss in the first week of degradation for either Group A or B (Fig. 6). For Group A, statistically significant decreases in mass were detected only after Week 3; specifically 95.9±0.8% mass remained at Week 2, and by the end of Week 3 it had decreased to 93.0±1.8%. After the third week the mass began to decrease much more rapidly than it had in the first three weeks. There was only 82.7±2.5% and 68.6±4.1% mass remaining after four and six weeks of degradation, respectively. Finally at Week 8 the mass was only 38.3±3.1% of its original value. Group B, on the other hand, showed slow mass loss until Week 4 at which time it had 88.6±2.4% mass remaining. As in Group A, the mass loss accelerated with time; at Week 8, there was only 42.5±1.3% mass remaining.

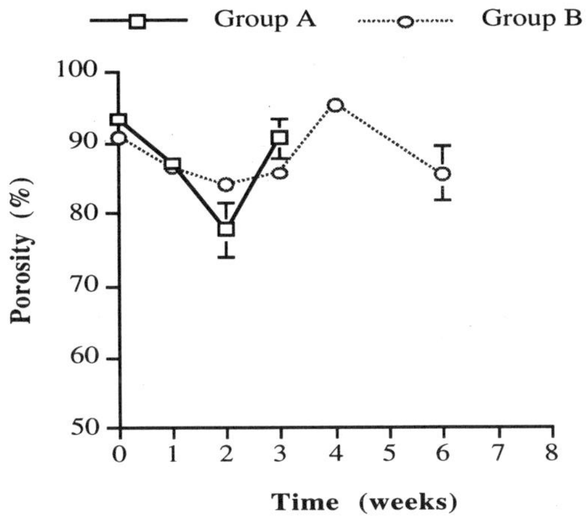

Fig. 5 - *Effects of degradation on the percent porosity of the biodegradable scaffolds. The porosity first decreased up to two weeks and then increased.*

Molecular Weight

Both groups exhibited almost identical trends in the decrease in molecular weight. Unlike the loss in mass, the molecular weight commenced to decrease instantaneously upon start of degradation and fell precipitously until Week 4 for both groups (Fig. 7); for example, at Week 4, Group A had only 31.3±1.2% of its original molecular weight remaining. However, there were no significant changes in molecular weight between Weeks 4 and 8 for either group.

Polydispersity

The polydispersity values are shown in Fig. 8. Group A showed a statistically significant dip in polydispersity over the first three weeks: 1.88±0.08 at t=0 and 1.11±0.18 at t=3 weeks. However by Week 4 the polydispersity had increased to 1.94±0.16. Group B showed only minimal changes in the polydispersity value over eight weeks.

Mechanical Properties

At t = 0 the elastic modulus (E) was 0.03±0.01 MPa for the Group A implants (Fig. 9). After one week of degradation there was a significant increase in stiffness and the value of E was 0.11±0.05 MPa. Subsequently the specimens became softer and at Week 2 E was 0.05±0.03 MPa. Beyond that time point, the implants had undergone too many structural and mechanical changes to be tested accurately. Group B specimens were significantly stiffer than Group A implants at t = 0; the initial stiffness of Group B specimens was 0.23±0.06 MPa. This value slightly increased through Week 3 and then fell to 0.16±0.08 MPa in the fourth week.

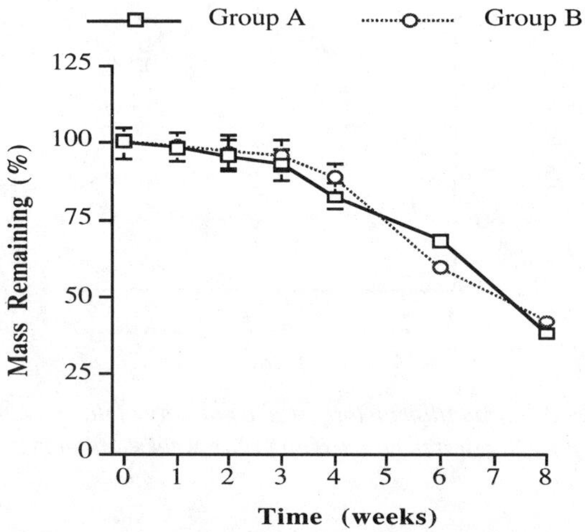

Fig. 6 - *Percent mass remaining as a function of degradation time. The mass loss is slow in the beginning.*

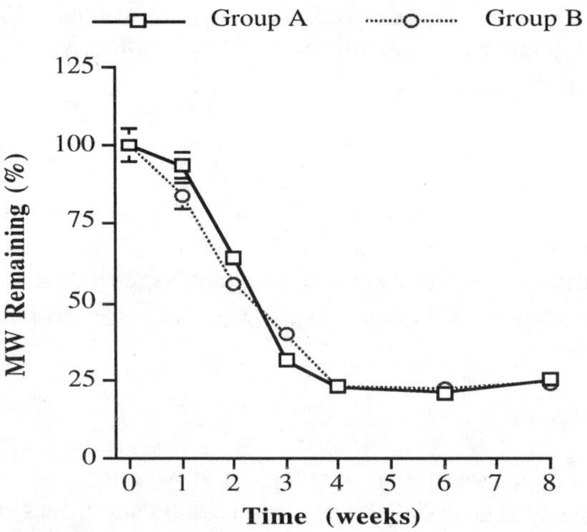

Fig. 7 - *Effects of hydrolytic degradation on the weight-average molecular weight (MW) of the polylactic acid - polyglycolic acid copolymer as a function of time. There were no significant differences between Groups A and B.*

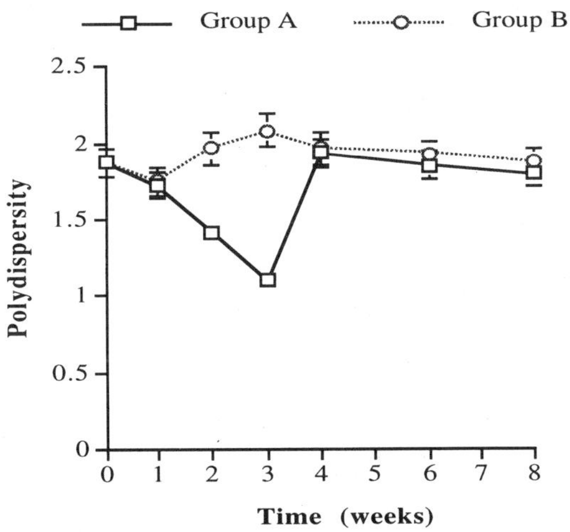

Fig. 8 - *Changes in polydispersity of the polymer as a function of degradation time.*

Size and Morphology

The change in morphology was similar for Groups A and B over the degradation time evaluated in this study. Scaffolds in both groups decreased in size over the first weeks of degradation. At t=3 weeks the diameter and height of the Group A implants had decreased to 71.3±6.8% and 63.2±13.3% of their initial values, respectively. This initial loss of height and diameter was followed by a significant increase in these dimensions. At Week 4 the diameter and height were 200.7±10.6% and 123.3±20.2% of their initial values, respectively, for Group A. Similar swelling occurred during Week 5 of degradation in Group B. Scanning electron micrographs of Group A specimens at Week 3 (before swelling) and at Week 4 (after swelling) are shown in Figures 10a and 10b. The development of micropores can be discerned at Week 4, which is indicative of swelling. After the swelling the implants once again began to decrease in size.

Discussion

The vibrating-particle technique described in this study yields scaffolds that have higher permeability compared to the salt-leaching technique (Table 1). This new technique also yields specimens without a polymeric film on one end, thus eliminating the need for its removal. Lastly, the pores are more evenly distributed throughout the scaffold compared to the salt-leaching technique. These attributes may make the new scaffold more receptive to cell infiltration and the formation of tissue.

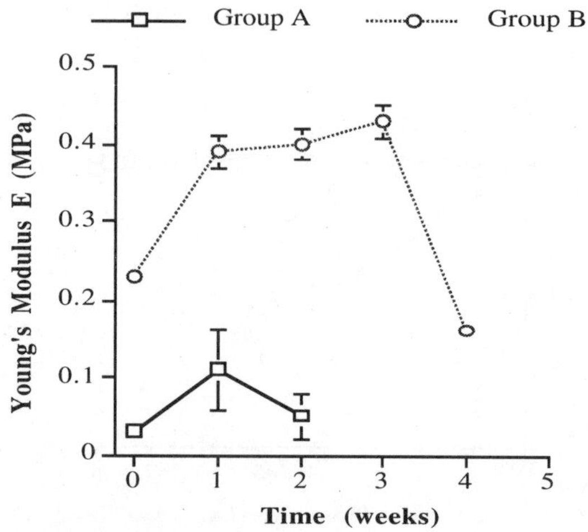

Fig. 9 - *Effects of degradation on the elastic modulus of the scaffold. The scaffolds exhibit an initial increase in stiffness.*

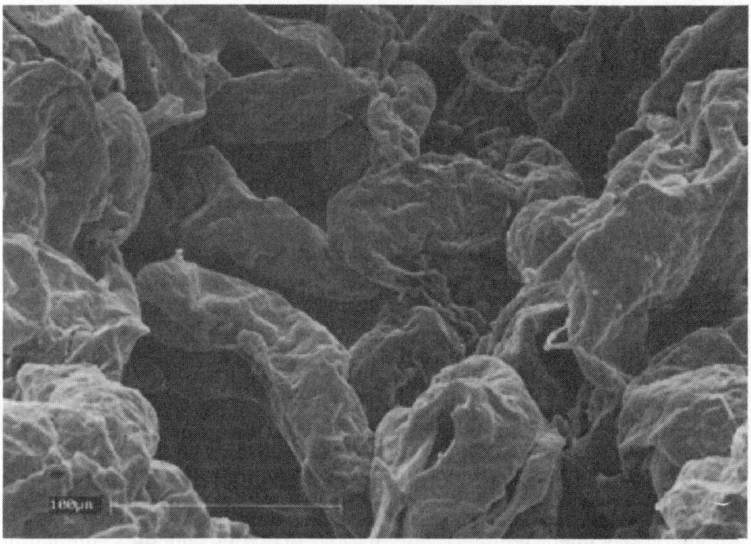

Fig. 10a – *Micrographs of scaffolds at (a) Week 3 – prior to swelling.*

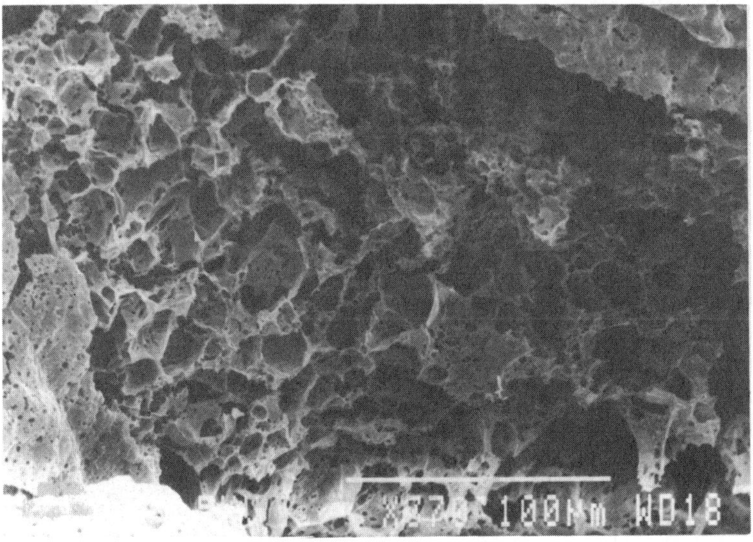

Fig. 10b – *Micrographs of scaffolds at Week 4 – after swelling. The Week 4 scaffold exhibits additional microstructure and the formation of new micropores.*

The specimens in Group B had a permeability which was approximately ten times higher compared to Group A at t=0. However, this difference in permeability was not reflected in the difference in porosity, which was in the range of 90.8 to 93.1% for the two groups. Furthermore, changes in the porosity and permeability as a function of degradation time did not exhibit similar trends (Figs. 4 and 5) indicating that permeability and porosity are not always coupled. Permeability is a measure of the ease with which a fluid can traverse through a structure. Porosity, on the other hand, is an indicator of the amount of void space within the structure. Although, intuitively it would appear that higher porosity should result in higher permeability, such is not always the case. For instance, a highly porous structure may have closed pores and hence very low permeability. In the present study, however, the pores were all interconnected as determined by inspection using scanning electron microscopy. It should be noted that pore size, pore orientation and tortuosity may also play a significant role in determining permeability.

Earlier, it has been shown by our laboratory that permeability and porosity can significantly influence the rate of degradation of biodegradable PLG implants [*3*]. It was determined that high porosity implants degraded significantly more slowly compared to low porosity specimens, possibly due to effects of autocatalysis. In the present study, the rates of degradation (measured in terms of loss in mass and molecular weight) for specimens from the two test groups exhibited very similar trends. This result is in agreement with our previous study [*3*], because the porosity of specimens in Groups A and B were comparable; on the other hand, there was a significant difference in the permeability. Thus, it may be inferred that this difference in permeability was not large enough to affect the degradation. It is possible that there is a threshold permeability above which autocatalysis is not an issue and the rate of degradation is virtually independent of the permeability.

The porosity of the specimens in both Groups A and B decreased initially for two weeks (Fig. 5). This decrease may be a reflection of the scaffold structure initially contracting, perhaps due to the recoil of polymeric molecular chains locked in stretched conformations as a result of the energy provided by the vibration during the solvent evaporation and polymer precipitation process. The plasticizing effect provided by water molecules would provide the requisite flexibility to the molecular chains to return to their preferred positions. Upon longer periods of immersion, the water molecules would induce swelling in the polymer. The increase in separation between the PLG molecular chains during swelling would result in a reduction of secondary intermolecular bonding forces. Such a loss of secondary bond interactions may then cause the structure to soften [*8*]. Indeed, a decrease in mechanical stiffness was observed for both Groups A and B after an initial two to three weeks. The changes in gross morphology and size due to degradation follow this hypothesis. There was an initial loss of size but not mass, supporting the idea that the scaffold structure was contracting as the implant's polymeric chains returned to their favored conformations. A swelling phenomenon was subsequently observed, in agreement with our hypothesis.

Prior to degradation, the stiffness of Group B implants was approximately 7.6 times greater compared to Group A specimens. As the same polymer was used for the fabrication of the two groups, this large difference in stiffness can only be attributed to changes in the fabrication technique, which used approximately 6.2 times more polymer for Group B; the salt to polymer ratio for Groups A and B was 40:1 and 14:1 respectively. The porosities of the two groups, however, did not exhibit large differences. Possibly due to reasons related to chain recoil, the stiffness, measured in terms of elastic modulus, initially increased for both groups. Following this initial increase, stiffness decreased for both groups, although, specimens in Group B appeared to retain their mechanical properties longer than Group A. The initial gain and subsequent loss of mechanical stiffness by the implant is similar to that reported in an earlier study by Athanasiou et al. [*3*].

The changes in stiffness as a function of degradation time appeared to follow a trend opposite to that exhibited by the porosity (Figs. 5 and 9). The porosity of the specimens in both groups first decreased and then increased. A decrease in porosity would suggest a more dense construct with enhanced mechanical properties. Implants designed as scaffolds for cartilage or bone repair would ideally be expected to provide support for 8 to 12 weeks to permit the growth of neo-tissue. In such a case, specimens in Group B would be expected to fare better as they retain their mechanical strength longer compared to Group A scaffolds.

The rates of mass and molecular weight loss in this study were compared to assess if the new fabrication technique caused any changes. However, the specimens in both groups exhibited accelerated molecular weight loss compared to mass loss, which is normal for polymers that undergo bulk degradation. As detailed earlier by Agrawal et al. [*9,10*] the polymeric chains need to be substantially reduced in size by hydrolysis before they can freely diffuse out of the specimen matrix and contribute to mass loss. In an earlier paper, Thompson et al. [*11*] reported that the mass of the biodegradable porous PLG scaffolds did not significantly decrease over the first three weeks *in vitro,* although the molecular weight decreased; in the fourth week, mass began to rapidly decrease.

The polydispersity of the polymer for the two groups did not follow similar trends as a function of degradation time (Fig. 8). Unlike Group B, Group A showed a significant decrease in polydispersity over the first three weeks. Such a decrease could be a manifestation of preferential hydrolysis of the longer or shorter molecular chains in the polymer. A more likely scenario, however, is that the short-chain degradation products were able to diffuse out of the system at a rapid rate while the longer chains remained trapped in the matrix. As seen in Fig. 8, the polydispersity value for Group A approaches unity by Week 3 thereby indicating that the variation in chain size is decreasing and most of the remaining chains are similar in size. Upon further degradation by Week 4, chains of all sizes may be able to diffuse out evenly, leaving behind a more random distribution of chain sizes, thereby returning the polydispersity close to its original value. This agrees with the observation that the rate of loss of mass increased between Weeks 3 and 4. On the other hand, the scaffolds from Group B showed steady values for polydispersity. This difference in behavior between the two groups may be related to the higher permeability of Group B specimens, although the exact reason is not clear.

In summary, this study used a new technique to fabricate biodegradable scaffolds; this method eliminated some problems associated with the salt-leaching technique, and the resulting scaffolds exhibited extremely high porosity and permeability. Although the high permeability would certainly be expected to be advantageous for the inflow of nutrients or growth factors, and the effusion of waste products, it was not found to affect the rate of degradation. The study also demonstrated that the permeability of a scaffold can vary dramatically without significant changes in the corresponding porosity. Thus, measurement of scaffold porosity alone may not be sufficient to gauge its efficacy. Lastly, this study established that the vibrating particle technique introduced here can yield scaffolds that not only have high porosity and permeability but also retain their mechanical properties for a significant period of time.

References

[1] Freed, L. E., Vunjak-Novakovic, G., Biron, R. J., Eagles, D. B., Lesnoy, D. C., Barlow, S. K., and Langer, R., "Biodegradable Polymer Scaffolds for Tissue Engineering." *Bio/Technology*, 12, 1994, p. 689.

[2] Freed, L. E., Vunjak-Novakovic, G., and Langer, R., "Cultivation of Cell-Polymer Cartilage Implants in Bioreactors." *Journal of Cellular Biochemistry*, 51, 1993, p. 257.

[3] Athanasiou, K. A., Schmitz, J. P., and Agrawal, C. M., "The Effects of Porosity on In Vitro Degradation of Polylactic Acid-Polyglycolic Acid Implants Used in Repair of Articular Cartilage." *Tissue Engineering*, 4(1), 1998, p. 53.

[4] Agrawal, C. M., Athanasiou, K. A., and Heckman, J. D., "Biodegradable PLA-PGA Polymers for Tissue Engineering in Orthopaedics, in Porous Materials for Tissue Engineering," D-M. Liu and V. Dixit, Eds. Trans Tech Publications Inc., Switzerland, 1997.

[5] Mikos, A. G., Sarakinos, G., Leite, S. M., Vacanti, J. P., and Langer, R., "Laminated Three-Dimensional Biodegradable Foams for Use in Tissue Engineering." *Biomaterials*, 14(5), 1993, p. 323.

[6] Spain, T. L., Agrawal, C. M., and Athanasiou, K. A., "A New Technique to Extend the Useful Life of a Biodegradable Cartilage Implant." *Tissue Engineering*, 4(4), 1998, p. 343.

[7] Singhal, A. R., Agrawal, C. M., and Athanasiou, K. A., "Salient Degradation Features of a 50:50 PLA/PGA Scaffold for Tissue Engineering." *Tissue Engineering*, 2, 1996, p. 197.

[8] Callister, W. D. Jr., "Corrosion and Degradation of Materials, in Materials Science and Engineering: An Introduction." John Wiley & Sons Inc., New York, 1991, p. 596.

[9] Agrawal, C. M., Niederaurer, G. G., Micallef, D. M., and Athanasiou, K. A., "The Use of PLA-PGA Polymers in Orthopaedics." *Encyclopedic Handbook of Biomaterials and Bioengineering*, 2, 1995, p. 1055.

[10] Agrawal, C. M., Huang, D., Schmitz, J. P., and Athanasiou, K. A., "Elevated Temperature Degradation of a 50:50 Copolymer of PLA-PGA." *Tissue Engineering*, 3(4), 1997, p. 345.

[11] Thompson, D. E., Agrawal, C. M., and Athanasiou, K. A., "The Effects of Dynamic Compressive Loading on Biodegradable Implants of 50-50% Polylactic Acid-Polyglycolic Acid." *Tissue Engineering*, 2(1), 1996, p. 61.

Karen J. L. Burg,[1] Catherine E. Austin,[2] and Jeanene P. Swiggett[2]

Modulation of Pore Topography of Tissue Engineering Constructs

---

Reference: Burg, K. J. L., Austin, C. E., Swiggett, J. P., "**Modulation of Pore Topography of Tissue Engineering Constructs**," *Synthetic Bioabsorbable Polymers for Implants, ASTM STP1396*, C. M. Agrawal, J. E. Parr, and S. T. Lin, Eds., American Society for Testing and Materials, West Conshohocken, PA, 2000.

Abstract: Absorbable materials can be used in tissue engineering to provide a porous template into which cells can be dispersed. The template not only serves as the delivery vehicle for implantation, but it also provides the form that the developing tissue will eventually take. The physicochemical properties of the material influence the development of cells within the template. This preliminary study assessed the effect of two template processing techniques on cellular attachment using sheep uterus smooth muscle cells and poly-l-lactide constructs. The results demonstrate that porogen selection in solvent cast, particulate-leached templates can radically change cellular attachment behavior.

Keywords: absorbable, porogen, porosity, tissue engineering

Introduction

Absorbable polymers are used in tissue engineering as temporary, porous constructs to guide developing tissue [*1-4*]. The molecular structure of the material is important, but the topography is equally so. The topography of the scaffold, specifically the interconnectivity of pores, pore shapes, and surface texture, largely influences the adhesion and proliferation of cells throughout the entire material volume [*5, 6*]. This is important to the long-term success of the implant, since the goal is to replace the biomaterial eventually through infiltration of tissue. The *in vivo* cellular response to the material is dictated by the features of the material; thus, depending on the material design, an array of fibrotic response levels can be induced [*7, 8*]. The quality and function of the developing tissue can therefore vary widely with biomaterial type. Absorbable, porous tissue engineering scaffolds are complex. In addition to the dynamic outer surface, the dynamic inner surface is also exposed and will immediately interact with cells.

There are many methods of manufacturing porous, absorbable scaffolds [*4, 9*]; one common mode of processing a porous construct is by solid dispersion [*10*], i.e., incorporating a solid, leachable phase with the polymeric phase. Traditional particulate

---

[1]Assistant professor, Department of Bioengineering, Clemson University, 501 Rhodes Engineering Research Center, Clemson, SC 29634-0905

[2]Laboratory technician II and senior research analyst, respectively, Department of General Surgery Research, Carolinas Medical Center, 406 Cannon, P.O. Box 32861, Charlotte, NC 28232-2861.

leaching techniques use sodium chloride (NaCl; "salt") as the particulate or porogen, which produces a sharp, cubic lattice. Previous work [*5, 6*] with poly-l-lactide has shown that glucose may be used similarly as a porogen, resulting in a much smoother pore structure and enhanced cellular adhesion, as judged by migration of cells within the construct as well as metabolic and biochemical behavior. The focus of this work was to expand this preliminary work, observing the behavior of cells over a time course study in a poly-l-lactide system.

Materials and Methods

Polymer

Polylactide (PLLA) disc matrices (270 000 daltons weight average molecular weight and 68% crystallinity, PURAC Biochem; Gorinchem, The Netherlands), 3-mm thickness and 13-mm diameter, were processed according to a standard solid dispersion technique [*1*] using six different porogen types, four salts and two sugars, to demonstrate the efficacy of porogen variability in morphology manipulation. Upon successful demonstration of this point, 21 PLLA discs were manufactured using sodium chloride porogen and 21 PLLA discs were manufactured using glucose porogen to yield constructs of approximately 96% porosity. All discs were ethanol treated, then soaked in Smooth Muscle Basal Medium prior to cell culture.

Cell Culture

Serial cultures of sheep uterus smooth muscle cells (USMC) were established from dispersion culture [*11*]. The smooth muscle cells were grown in Smooth Muscle Basal Medium supplemented with SMGM2 (Clonetics; San Diego, CA) and incubated in a 5% carbon dioxide, humidified environment. The cells were serially cultured to passage 9, at which time the cells were washed with phosphate buffered saline (Sigma; St. Louis, MO) and resuspended at 1×10^7 cells/ml in media. Six 150-mL paddle stir flasks (Kontes; Vineland, NJ), hereafter referred to as "experimental," were each loaded with 1×10^7 cells and 100 ml media. Three experimental flasks were loaded with glucose leached discs (GL), and three were loaded with salt leached discs (SL), five discs per flask. Two additional flasks, labeled "controls," were loaded with 100 mL media and six discs each. One control flask contained GL discs and the other contained SL discs. All flasks were incubated at 37 °C and allowed to stir at 25 rpm for the remainder of the study. Media was changed at regular intervals.

Analyses

One experimental flask for each disc type was retrieved after 2, 6, and 16 days incubation. Three discs from each flask were used for metabolic activity assays, and two were used for viability testing and confocal image analysis. Two discs from each control flask were removed at each time point for metabolic activity and viability analyses, respectively. Two samples of 6-mm diameter were punched from each disc using a biopsy punch (Baker Cummins; Miami, FL), representative of the central portion and the edge portion of the disc. Media from all flasks was analyzed at each time point using a YSI 2300 Stat/L-lactate analyzer (Yellow Springs Instrument Co.; Yellow Springs, OH) to assess lactic acid and glucose concentrations in each.

Viability Testing and Confocal Microscopy - A viability/cytotoxicity kit (Molecular Probes; Eugene, OR) was used to label the cells fluorescently and then make qualitative observations using an Olympus IX 70 inverted microscope with an IX FLA fluorescence observation attachment (Olympus America Inc; Melville, NY). Live cells are distinguished by a green fluorescence (excitation wavelength 495 nm and emission wavelength 515 nm). Dead cells were distinguished by a red fluorescence with an excitation wavelength of 495 nm and an emission wavelength of 635 nm. The discs were scanned using a Leica TCS SP (Leica Microsystems; Heidelberg, Germany) confocal microscope. The top plane of each disc was brought into focus using light microscopy, then the depth of cellular penetration into the matrix was determined, and this thickness was scanned in dual color confocal mode, capturing 16 even slices in the vertical direction. These 16 images were overlaid into one two-dimensional composite image and captured in a file. A single image of the top plane in each disc was also scanned and captured. All images were captured at 25× magnification. Measurements were taken on the six-day samples to determine the depth of penetration of cellular growth.

Metabolic Acitivity - The metabolic activity in the discs was assessed using an MTT (3-[4,5-Dimethylthiazol-2]-2,5-diphenyltetrazolium bromide) assay. A solution of 0.5 mg/mL MTT was made in 2% fetal bovine serum in media, and 1 mL was applied to each disc. The discs were incubated at 37 °C for 1 hour on a shaker plate, rinsed twice with phosphate buffered saline, then soaked in 1 mL of isopropanol for 15 minutes at 37 °C for extraction. Extractions were repeated to a complete depletion of blue coloration in the discs. Two hundred microliters from each extraction was transferred to a 96 well plate and read at 540 nm using a Universal Microplate Reader EL800 (BIO-TEK Instruments, Inc.; Winooski, VT).

Results and Discussion

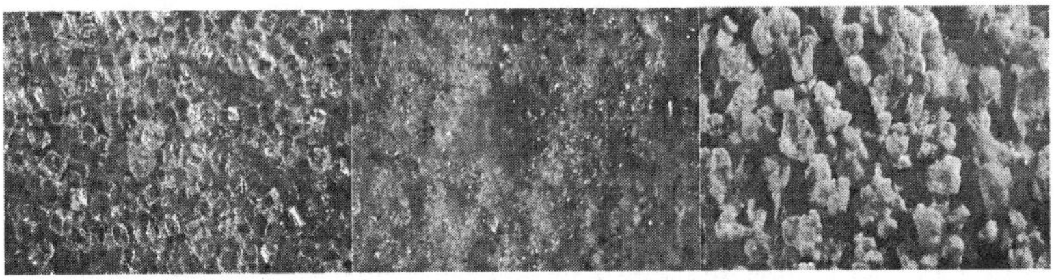

a b c

FIG. 1-*Differing polylactide morphologies as formed using* (a) *sodium chloride,* (b) *potassium phosphate, and* (c) *sodium phosphate. Stereomicroscopy at 20 times magnification.*

Figures 1a, 1b, and 1c show different polymeric matrices, including sodium phosphate, sodium chloride, and potassium phosphate which have been successfully formed by solvent casting and particulate leaching, and which all have extremely different pore morphologies. The concept of solvent casting and particulate leaching is by no means a new technique; rather, it was developed in the packaging industry and has been more recently applied to absorbable processing with a specific emphasis on tissue engineering. Careful selection of pore size is a standard in the filter industry, where the pore size is critical to the selectivity of a given membrane. Pore topography has been cited as a key player in modulating tissue ingrowth of porous implants, and thus a key factor in their longterm stability. It is these core studies that have lead to the interest in customizing pore topography and size in tissue engineered, three-dimensional constructs in order to provide both site specificity and ingrowth control. All discs shown in Figure 1 formed cohesive, three-dimensional, porous constructs of varying pore morphology. The resultant pore morphologies were directly related to the porogen shape and, therefore, varied radically with crystal structure. It is hypothesized, based on prior literature, that this will have a profound influence on cellular attachment [*5, 6*]; thus, this work has led to the development of migration assays specific to three-dimensional porous constructs. Previous work by Burg and coworkers assessed similar polylactide matrices with rat aortic smooth muscle cells and found that glucose porogen significantly enhanced cellular proliferation over a six-day time period. This past study did not examine cellular attachment and/or growth at earlier time points; therefore, the results of the present study including the relatively superior results of the sodium chloride constructs after a day in culture were not observed. It therefore reinforces the need for carefully selecting the cellular concentration and seeding time prior to implantation. The preliminary studies discussed in this paper, addressing glucose and salt as porogens suggest that the porogen selection is essential to the development of appropriate tissue and subsequent integration post-implantation.

Viability Testing and Confocal Microscopy

The SL pore structure was visible when illuminated by the laser light (Figure 2), emitted light in the 580 to 700 nm range, whereas the GL structure is not clearly defined. This was most likely due to residual salt in the system, either a direct image of sodium chloride autofluorescence or an image of nonviable cells that were affected by the sodium chloride presence. It is unlikely that the processing changed the polymeric physicochemical features to cause this effect, although that possibility certainly can not be ruled out. To assess this further, salt crystals and glucose crystals, placed in saline solution, were both scanned to observe autofluorescence. The salt crystals do indeed fluoresce in laser light, as can be noted from Figure 3a. Figure 3b shows glucose crystals that were clearly visible; the clarity of this picture diminishes with dissolution of the crystals in solution. This phenomenon is quite important since, according to earlier studies [*5*], all measurable quantities of salt and glucose are removed from the discs during processing. Clearly, small amounts of recrystallization during the drying process can radically change the quality of the system.

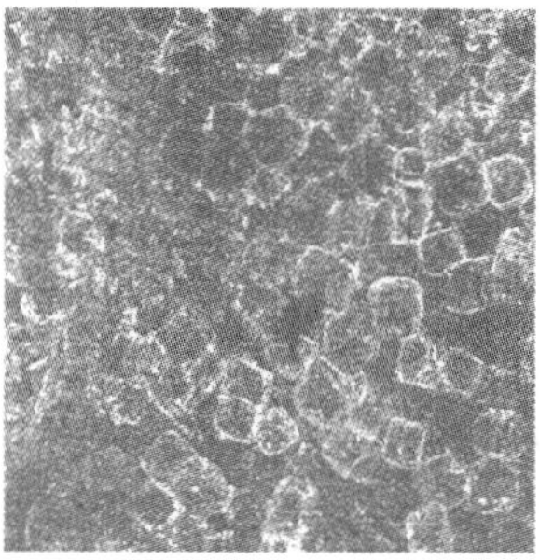

FIG. 2-*SL pore structure at 25 times magnification.*

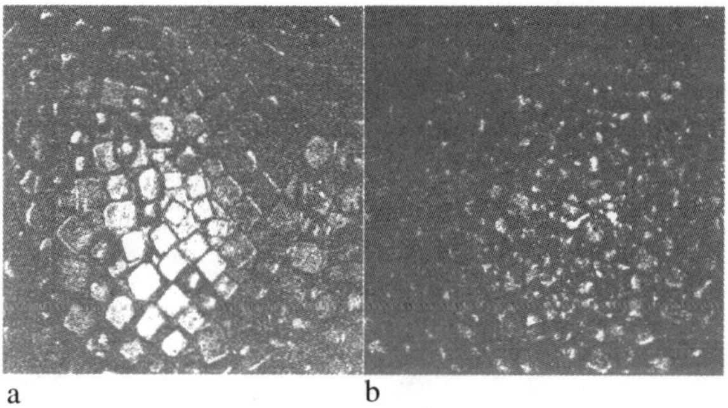

FIG. 3 - *Confocal microscopy showing* (a) *sodium chloride fluorescence and* (b) *glucose.*

At time 1, the surface of the GL discs, both at the edge and in the center, showed minimal cell growth, as compared with the SL structures which had cellular growth at the edges only. Figure 4 demonstrates the surface view of the GL and SL edges, and the patchier appearance of cells within the SL disc. Scanning into the polymer and compiling these sections showed that the GL discs had cellular ingrowth both at the center and edge regions to a depth of approximately 1 mm, though with diminished cellular concentration. The pore topography again was evident within the SL structure and not within the GL structure.

After six days incubation, the GL material had even cellular distribution across the face, both on the surface and up to a 1-mm depth, whereas the SL cellular distribution was sporadic at best. Figure 5 demonstrates the compiled images of 1-mm depth in both systems. The stir flask system, while an excellent system for smaller constructs such as beads, is not yet optimized for these larger porous constructs. After 16 days in this environment, the stir flask had begun to damage the polymers mechanically, so very little was seen in cellular growth as the outer layers were peeled away. Dead cells were also monitored, fluorescing in the 580 to 700nm range and were present in all cases. It was difficult to distinguish these using confocal microscopy due to the fluorescent features of the SL materials, therefore no conclusions can be drawn concerning nonviable cells within the pores.

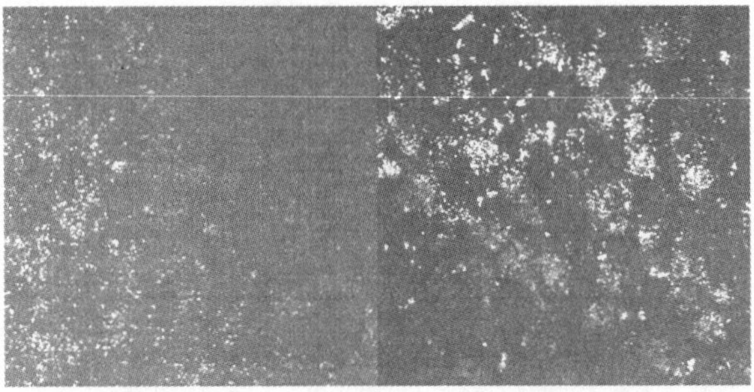

a b

FIG. 4-*White areas indicate areas of cellular growth in the edge regions of* (a) *GL and* (b) *SL disc surfaces, taken at 25 times magnification after two days culture.*

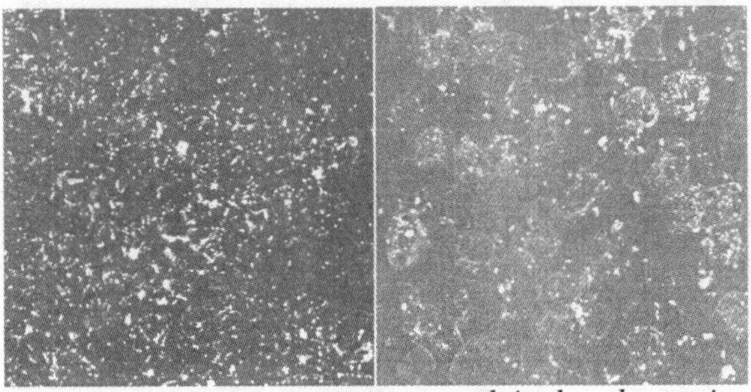

FIG. 5- *White areas indicate areas of cellular growth in the edge regions of* (a) *GL and* (b) *SL discs, taken at 25 times magnification after 6 days culture.*

Metabolic Activity and Glucose/Lactic Acid Analysis

The SL discs, both controls and experimental, were more yellow, perhaps due to sodium ions in the media. The cumulative lactic acid release and glucose uptake is plotted in Figure 6. There was no leached glucose as determined by the YSI measurements of the controls, reinforcing observations from earlier studies [5]. The cumulative lactic acid release did not differ between the sodium chloride control and the glucose control. There was an accumulation of lactic acid in both control systems, indicating similar degradation of the two polymer types. The experimental systems were not significantly different after two or six days; however, after 16 days the glucose system expressed a larger lactic acid release.

Measurements of glucose remaining in the media demonstrated that the control media showed identical accumulation patterns and the experimental systems a significantly ($p < 0.05$) higher glucose uptake in the SL system. It is hypothesized that these observations are attributed in part to the residual glucose on the constructs. If the cells used this recrystallized glucose as their energy source, the media levels of glucose would not be consumed as quickly. The glucose measurements account for dissolved glucose, hence this value in the GL system would remain relatively stable over time with an additional presence of crystallized glucose. Metabolic activity, however, was much higher in the

GL discs than in the SL discs after two days' incubation but not significantly different after six or sixteen days. Level of metabolic activity is not necessarily an indicator of cellular number, since a large number of cells with low metabolic activity might have equivalent activity to a low number of cells with high metabolic activity. Metabolic activity can be indicative of the cellular state as to an adhesion or proliferation state. Presence of metabolic activity simply demonstrates that the cells are not in a quiescent state; further biochemical analyses would be needed to elucidate reasons for differences in metabolic activity levels. The lower MTT values after two days incubation may be indicative of the proximity of cells, largely aggregates, with one another in the SL material, thus diminishing the cellular activities. It does not appear, qualitatively, to be due to diminished cellular number.

It could be argued that; since, residual porogens are critical to cellular behavior, then it would be advantageous to remove them completely. This, however, is not feasible by standard leaching techniques since the requisite time to do so would cause mechanical degradation of the polylactide structure via hydrolysis. The simpler method is to select porogens that, in residual quantity, will enhance cellular growth and thus be an integral component in the absorbable construct and subsequent development of tissue.

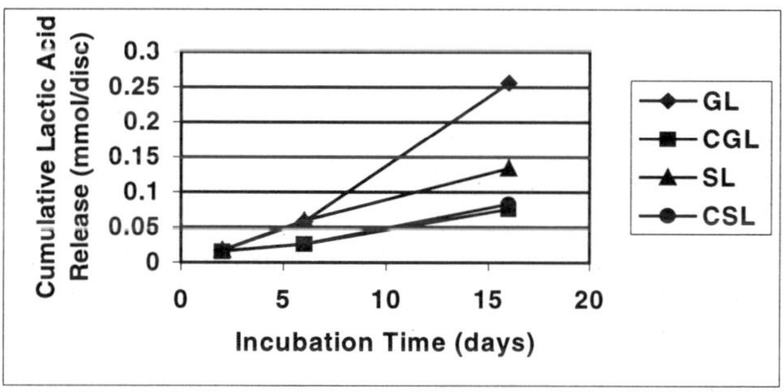

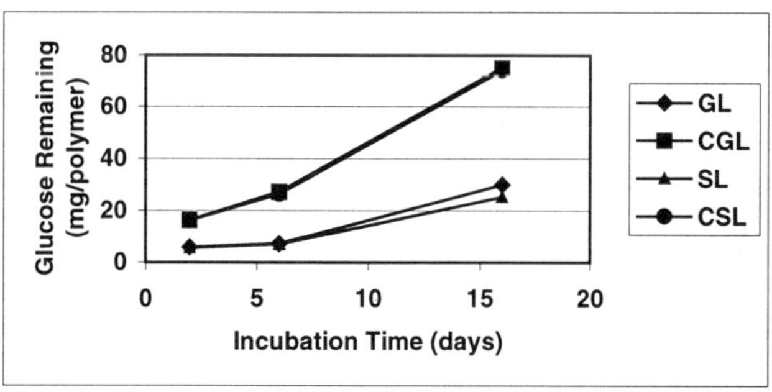

FIG. 6- *Metabolic activity with incubation time including* (a) *cumulative lactic acid release and* (b) *cumulative glucose amounts remaining, "C" indicates control polymers. Standard error bars are smaller than the data points and thus are not visible.*

Conclusions

The GL discs caused enhanced cellular proliferation after a culture time of six days as compared with SL discs. The initial attachment of cells occurred much faster in the SL system; however, the result was the development of a low concentration of aggregates with time. Porogen selection is critical to cellular behavior; small residual amounts post-processing can influence cellular development as well. It will be of future interest to conduct a more detailed study investigating increased disc numbers using an optimized stir flask system.

References

[1] Freed, L. E., Marquis, J. C., Nohria, A., Emmanual, J., Mikos, A. G., and Langer, R., "Neocartilage Formation In Vitro And In Vivo Using Cells Cultured On Synthetic Biodegradable Polymers," *Journal of Biomedical Materials Research,* Vol. 27, 1993, pp. 11-23.

[2] Cima, L. G., Vacanti, J. P., Vacanti, C., Ingber, D., Mooney, D., and Langer, R., "Tissue Engineering By Cell Transplantation Using Degradable Polymer Substrates," *Journal of Biomechanical Engineering*, Vol. 113, No. 2, 1991, pp. 143-151.

[3] Mikos, A. G., Sarakinos, G., Leite, S. M., Vacanti, J. P., and Langer, R., "Laminated Three-Dimensional Biodegradable Foams For Use In Tissue Engineering," *Biomaterials*, Vol. 14, No. 5, 1993, pp. 323-330.

[4] Burg, K. J. L. and Shalaby, S. W., "Bioabsorbable Polymers," *The Polymeric Materials Encyclopedia,* J. Salamone, Ed., CRC Press, Boca Raton, FL, 1996, pp. 535-538.

[5] Burg, K. J. L., Mikos, A. G., Beiler, R. J., Culberson, C. R., Greene, K. G., Loebsack, A. B., Roland, W. D., Wyatt, S., Halberstadt, C. R., Holder, W. D., Jr., and Burg, T. C., "Particulate Selection And Importance To Cell Adhesion In Solvent-Cast, Particulate-Leached Polymeric Constructs," *Transactions of the 25th Annual Meeting of the Society for Biomaterials*, May 1999.

[6] Holy, C. E., Dang, S. M., Davies, J. E., and Shoichet, M. S., "In Vitro Degradation Of A Novel Poly(Lactide-Co-Glycolide) 75/25 Foam," *Biomaterials*, Vol. 20, 1999, pp. 1177-1185.

[7] den Braber, E. T., de Ruijter, J. E., Ginsel, L. A., von Recum, A. F., and Jansen, J. A., "Quantitative Analysis Of Fibroblast Morphology On Microgrooved Surfaces With Various Groove And Ridge Dimensions," *Biomaterials,* Vol. 17, No. 21, 1996, pp. 2037-2044.

[8] von Recum, A. F., Opitz, H., and Wu, E., "Collagen Types I and III at the Implant/Tissue Interface," *Journal of Biomedical Materials Research*, Vol. 27, No. 6, 1993, pp. 757-761.

[9] Roweton, S. L., "A New Approach To The Formation Of Tailored Microcellular Foams And Microtextured Surfaces Of Absorbable And Non-Absorbable Thermoplastic Biomaterials," *Master of Science Thesis*, Department of Bioengineering, Clemson University, 1994.

[10] Mikos, A. G., Thorsen, A. J., Czerwonka, L. A., Bao, Y., and Langer, R., "Preparation And Characterization Of Poly(L-Lactic Acid) Foams," *Polymer,* Vol. 35, 1994, pp. 1068-1077.

[11] Holder, W. D. Jr., Gruber, H. E., Roland, W. D., Moore, A. L., Culberson, C. R., Loebsack, A. B., Burg, K. J. L., and Mooney, D. J., "Increased Vascularization And Heterogeneity Of Vascular Structures Occurring In Polyglycolide Matrices Containing Aortic Endothelial Cells Implanted In The Rat," *Tissue Engineering*, 3(2):149-160, Summer 1997.

Michael A. Slivka,[1] Neil C. Leatherbury,[1] Kris Kieswetter,[2] and Gabriele G. Niederauer[1]

In Vitro Compression Testing of Fiber-Reinforced, Bioabsorbable, Porous Implants

Reference: Slivka, M. A., Leatherbury, N. C., Kieswetter, K., and Niederauer, G. G., "***In Vitro* Compression Testing of Fiber-Reinforced, Bioabsorbable, Porous Implants**," *Synthetic Bioabsorbable Polymers for Implants, ASTM STP 1396,* C. M. Agrawal, J. E. Parr, and S. T. Lin, Eds., American Society for Testing and Materials, West Conshohocken, PA, 2000.

Abstract: Proper *in vitro* mechanical testing of medical devices requires consideration of many factors, including environmental conditions, implant characteristics, and nature of the test method. In this study, parallel plate compression testing of porous specimens composed of 75:25 poly(D,L-lactide-co-glycolide) reinforced with short polyglycolide fibers was used to show the effect of many factors on the compressive modulus and yield strength. Compressive properties were dramatically reduced when tested under physiological conditions (aqueous, 37 °C) versus ambient conditions. Predominant fiber alignment yielded superior properties when tested parallel to the fiber orientation, increasing the compressive properties proportionally with fiber content from 0% to 20%. With increasing strain rate over four orders of magnitude, compressive moduli increased logarithmically and yield strength increased in a semi-logarithmic fashion. After *in vitro* degradation for nine weeks, compressive properties decreased to less than 20% of their original values.

Keywords: compression, mechanical properties, fiber reinforcement, bioabsorbable, porous scaffold

Introduction

In recent years, tissue engineering has emerged as a field of intense study due in large part to the development of specialized scaffolds that act as permanent or temporary support structures for the ingrowth of new tissues. Certain demanding applications, such as repair of articular cartilage in the knee and bone void repair in long bones, require that the scaffold have high mechanical strength and stiffness close to that of the native tissue. Therefore, appropriate mechanical testing must be performed to assure that implants designed for such applications have the necessary properties to both support new tissue ingrowth and resist externally applied loads once implanted.

[1]Engineer, engineer, and director of research and development, respectively, OsteoBiologics, Inc., 12500 Network Suite 112, San Antonio, TX, 78249

[2]Principal research scientist, DPT Laboratories, 318 McCullough, San Antonio, TX, 78215.

A variety of scaffold constructs have been developed, depending on the type of application and the technique for achieving successful tissue repair. Highly porous (>90%), non-woven, fibrous scaffolds have proved very effective for applications where the new tissue is grown on the scaffold *in vitro* in a highly controlled environment and then implanted [*1-3*]. However, such a construct alone has negligible structural integrity to support *in situ* loading. Woven, low porosity (50%), carbon fiber scaffolds have been used clinically as a cartilage resurfacing implant [*4*], but are less accessible to tissue ingrowth and are not absorbable. A successful scaffold intended for immediate load bearing once implanted should have an open porous structure, made using materials that will be absorbed in the body over time, yet provide adequate mechanical properties.

Numerous open-pored, absorbable scaffolds have been proposed for tissue engineering applications. However, many researchers have not tested the mechanical properties of the scaffolds, and for those who have, the testing parameters and conditions varied greatly. Using dynamic mechanical analysis (DMA), the elastic and viscous components of the material stiffness are calculated as the storage modulus and loss modulus (or loss tangent), respectively, from the strain response to a sinusoidal applied force. Alternatively, a complex modulus may be calculated to incorporate the elastic and viscous components. Studies using ASTM Standard Test Method for Measuring the Dynamic Mechanical Properties of Plastics in Compression (D5024) on poly(L-lactide) (PLLA) scaffolds made using phase separation showed that the loss tangent increased when testing was done wet at 37 °C versus dry at 37 °C, reportedly due to fluid flow through the pores [*5*]. Poly(phosphoester) foams, also made using phase separation, were tested using DMA in phosphate buffer (pH 7.4) at 37 °C. After immersion for 3 weeks in the buffer at 37 °C, the complex modulus of the foams more than quadrupled and the loss tangent decreased by more than one-third, reportedly due to leaching of low molecular weight portions of the copolymer [*6*]. Alternatively, the changes could have occurred due to leaching of the napthalene or phenol solvents used to make the foams, since residual solvent analysis of the foams was not reported.

Like DMA, creep testing has been used to evaluate viscoelastic materials, such as polymeric scaffolds and connective tissues. Type I collagen sponges for articular cartilage repair were tested in creep using confined compression while submerged in a saline environment [*7*]. Results showed that the aggregate modulus (~0.08 MPa) was an order of magnitude lower than that for normal articular cartilage (~1 MPa) [*8*]. Compressive creep testing using ASTM Standard Test Methods for Tensile, Compressive, and Flexural Creep and Creep-Rupture of Plastics (D2990), under both dry and wet conditions at 37 °C, has also been used to evaluate PLLA foams made using phase separation. For a constant stress of 9.2 kPa held for 30 min, strains ranged from 0.1 for a 71% porous foam to 0.5 for an 87% porous foam [*5*], corresponding to a creep modulus of 0.45 and 0.092 MPa, respectively. Similar results were found for salt-leached PLLA, 85:15 poly(D,L-lactide-co-glycolide) (PLG), and 50:50 PLG using a creep stress of 9.5 kPa applied for 60 min at 37 °C. However, the 50:50 PLG had not reached an equilibrium strain after the 60 min creep time [*9*]. Creep testing with a porous indenter tip, which has been widely employed for testing articular cartilage [*8*], was used to evaluate 50:50 PLG scaffolds made using a vacuum expansion technique. Low (0%), moderate (33%), and high (75%) porosity scaffolds had Young's moduli of approximately 13, 4, and 12 MPa, respectively, when tested using a 0.5 mm diameter indenter tip applied with 0.083 N for one hour in saline at room temperature (environment assumed from cited reference) [*10*]. The same creep indentation technique and conditions were used to test 50% porous, 50:50 PLG scaffolds and "surface axial strain" was found to vary from 0.02 to 0.04. Upon *in vitro* degradation in phosphate buffered saline (PBS) at 37 °C, these implants became stiffer after two weeks, then softer after four weeks. Leaching of residual solvent was reported as the likeliest cause for initial stiffening of the scaffolds [*11*].

Simple compression testing using a constant rate of strain has also been used to test tissue engineering scaffolds. PLLA foams made using phase separation were tested at 0.5 mm min^{-1} (corresponding strain rate = 0.17 min^{-1}) under ambient conditions, and compressive modulus and yield strength were shown to increase when hydroxyapatite was used as reinforcement [*12*]. Salt-leached, polyurethane scaffolds were tested under ambient conditions at a loading rate of 2 mm min^{-1} and a strong positive correlation was shown between the scaffold density and Young's modulus [*13*]. Porogen-leached, 50:50 PLG scaffolds were tested at 1 mm min^{-1} using ASTM Standard Specification for Acrylic Bone (F451), corresponding to a strain rate of 0.07 min^{-1}, in a dry oven at 37 °C. A similar positive correlation was found between density and compressive modulus. The scaffolds were found to have inadequate mechanical properties and degradation rate (*in vitro*, PBS @ 37 °C) for trabecular bone repair [*14*]. Using the same testing method, the compressive properties of porogen-leached, 85:15 PLG scaffolds increased with the addition of short hydroxyapatite fibers at moderate porosity (47%). However, at high porosity, the reinforcement was not effective [*15*]. Salt-leached, poly(propylene fumarate)-based scaffolds were tested using the same parameters, except that testing was performed under ambient conditions, immediately after immersion in PBS at 37 °C without drying. *In vitro* degradation time in the PBS was then monitored for up to 12 weeks. Compressive modulus and yield strength increased during the first three weeks for three out of four of the formulations tested, then decreased, reportedly due to continued cross-linking of the polymer. Results for compressive modulus and strength were comparable to or greater than human trabecular bone [*16*].

Evaluation of the mechanical properties of absorbable scaffolds for tissue engineering applications is very difficult. The scaffolds are frequently sensitive to testing conditions such as temperature, environment, and strain rate. Water alone may cause viscous effects due to fluid flow within the pores, swelling of the polymeric material itself, and hydrolytic degradation. The porosity and physical dimensions of the test specimen may also affect the testing results. Furthermore, composite material scaffolds may have anisotropic mechanical properties. Therefore, the purpose of this study was to investigate the effects of various parameters and environmental conditions on the compressive modulus and yield strength of absorbable, fiber-reinforced, porous scaffolds recently proposed for tissue engineering applications [*17, 18*].

Materials and Methods

Manufacture of Porous Implants

Porous, composite implants were manufactured with a target volume porosity of 70%. The matrix polymer was 75:25 poly(D,L-lactide-co-glycolide) (PLG) (Boehringer Ingelheim, Ingelheim, Germany), with an inherent viscosity of 0.76 dL/g as received from the supplier. Fiber reinforcement was added using ~15 μm diameter, ~2.5 mm long, chopped polyglycolide (PGA) fibers (Albany International, Mansfield, MA) . Porosity and uniaxial fiber orientation were achieved using a process similar to published methods [*11, 19*], and summarized briefly as follows. The PLG was dissolved in acetone, the fibers were dispersed in ethanol, and the two were mixed to precipitate the PLG. The resulting composite gel was kneaded to disperse and preferentially orient the fibers, then shaped and placed in a long, cylindrical mold. The gel/mold was then placed under vacuum to foam the composite and heated to remove residual solvents. After curing, the porous composite was cut to a precise thickness using a wafering saw with a diamond-coated blade. After cutting, a core punch mounted in an arbor press was used to size the wafers to the specified diameter. Prior to using any implant specimen for the study, the residual levels of acetone and ethanol were verified as being below 100 ppm using gas chromatography.

Thermal Analysis

Thermal analysis of the PGA fibers alone and each of the porous scaffolds was conducted using a differential scanning calorimeter (DSC) to measure glass transition temperature. Specimens were heated at a rate of 10 °C/min from 0 to 250 °C to remove thermal history, then quenched cooled to 0 °C and heated a second time at 10 °C/min to 100 °C. From the thermogram obtained from the second run, the glass transition onset temperature was calculated.

Parallel Plate Compression Testing

Sample testing and analysis were performed using ASTM Test Method for Compressive Properties of Rigid Cellular Plastics (D1621) as a guide. Parallel plate compression testing was conducted using a uniaxial, electromechanical materials tester with a 500 N capacity, tension-compression load cell. The compressive modulus was calculated from the initial slope of the stress versus strain curve. For the fiber-reinforced scaffolds, a clear peak stress at yield was detected, and this was reported as the yield strength. For the scaffolds without fibers, a peak could not be clearly detected, so the yield stress at 1% offset was reported. Slack compensation and machine compliance were used to correct for errors in strain measurement. The faces of the stainless steel compression platens were circular with a diameter of 10 mm. Specimen dimensions were modified as appropriate for tissue engineering applications, i.e., bone and cartilage repair. Specimens had a height of 3.0 mm and diameter of 6.0 mm unless otherwise stated. All samples were tested in a direction parallel to the predominant orientation of the fibers unless otherwise stated. In conformance with D1621, all tests were performed at a strain rate of 0.10 min^{-1} unless otherwise stated. An environmental chamber was custom designed and built to allow for the test to be conducted in an aqueous bath maintained at 37 °C, to simulate general physiological conditions. All samples were tested at 37 °C in deionized water unless otherwise stated. For testing under ambient conditions, samples were left open in the laboratory for at least 24 hours prior to testing. Samples to be tested in aqueous environment were first infiltrated with the medium (water or PBS) by pulling vacuum on the sample. Adequate infiltration was achieved when the sample sank upon release of the vacuum. After infiltration, the samples were preconditioned in media at 37 °C for one hour prior to testing.

Testing Variables

To investigate the effect of environment on compressive properties, 10% PGA/PLG specimens were tested at one of three conditions: (1) ambient, (2) in deionized water at 37 °C, or (3) in phosphate buffered saline (PBS) at 37 °C (sample dimensions provided in Table 1). To determine the effect of fiber orientation, transversely isotropic specimens were tested either parallel or perpendicular to the predominant fiber alignment. Porous specimens were made with 0, 5, 10, 15, and 20% by weight fiber-reinforcement to study the effect on compressive properties. The dependence of strain rate (viscoelasticity) was determined by testing 10% PGA/PLG at 0.01, 0.1, 1, and 10 min^{-1}.

Specimens with 0, 10, and 20% fiber-reinforcement (5.0 mm height x 8.0 mm diameter) were subjected to *in vitro* degradation in PBS, supplemented with 0.01% w/v thimerosal as a preservative, and maintained at 37 °C. A 20x volume of PBS was used relative to the specimen volume, and was changed weekly. At time points of 0, 1, 2, 4, 6, and 9 weeks, samples were removed from the PBS, measured for height and diameter, immersed in the water bath at 37 °C, and tested.

Statistics

Each sample set consisted of five specimens. Mean and standard deviation were reported for compressive modulus and yield strength. Pairwise comparisons were made using the Student's t-test at a 95% confidence level. Linear regression was used to correlate mechanical properties with testing variables and the coefficient of determination (R^2) was reported.

Results and Discussion

From the mass, dimensions, and density of raw materials used in the scaffolds, the volume porosity was calculated to be 70% for both the PLG and 10% PGA/PLG scaffolds, but the 20% PGA/PLG was only 65%. At 20% fiber reinforcement, the precipitated composite gel became more difficult to knead and expand under vacuum, therefore reducing its final porosity.

Thermal analysis of PGA fibers and fiber-reinforced scaffolds revealed that the fibers alone had a glass transition temperature (T_g) of 33 °C, lower than the PLG scaffolds (50 °C), and also lower than human body temperature (37 °C). However, the T_g of the scaffolds did not change with increasing fiber content up to 20% by weight and was higher than body temperature. These results imply that the mechanical properties of the scaffolds should not be compromised at body temperature.

For 10% PGA/PLG specimens having identical dimensions, compressive modulus was 70 times greater and yield strength was 7 times greater when tested under ambient conditions than in water at 37 °C (Table 1). This dramatic difference is surprising considering that the T_g of the scaffold was well above the testing temperature. Most likely, the water is being absorbed into the polymer, causing a plasticizing effect. This, compounded with the increase in temperature, may explain the large difference in

Table 1 - *Compressive properties (mean ± standard deviation) of 10% PGA fiber-reinforced PLG, porous scaffolds measured under various test conditions (n=5, strain rate = 0.10 min^{-1}).*

Environmental Conditions	Test Direction[1]	Height mm	Diameter mm	Compressive Modulus MPa	Yield Strength MPa
Ambient	parallel	6.0	3.0	2 180 ± 145	14.1 ± 0.9
Water, 37 °C	parallel	6.0	3.0	31.7 ± 1.4	2.10 ± 0.50
Water, 37 °C	perp.	6.0	3.0	5.44 ± 0.63	0.257 ± 0.017
Water, 37 °C	parallel	8.0	5.0	44.4 ± 5.6	1.51 ± 0.15
PBS, 37 °C	parallel	8.0	5.0	44.8 ± 6.9	1.64 ± 0.20

[1]*relative to the predominant fiber orientation direction.*

compressive properties. As expected, the compressive properties did not change significantly ($p > 0.05$) when 10% PGA/PLG specimens having the same dimensions were tested in water at 37 °C versus in PBS at 37 °C (Table 1). Apparently, the plasticization is not affected by the salt concentration or buffering capacity of the aqueous solution.

However, when the 10% PGA/PLG scaffolds with different dimensions were tested under the same conditions, the compressive modulus and yield strength were statistically different ($p = 0.015$ and 0.023, respectively) (Table 1). Similar trends were reported for the compressive yield strength of 50:50 PLG foams tested with height:diameter aspect ratios between 2:1 and 1:2 [*14*]. Yielding of porous foams is generally caused when the pore walls buckle under the applied load. Pores on the periphery of the sample have less wall support, and therefore will buckle before interior pores. Hypothetically, as the diameter of the sample decreases (height:diameter increases), a higher percentage of the total pores are on the periphery of the foam, thus making the yield strength decrease.

As expected, compressive properties of 10% PGA/PLG specimens were significantly better when tested parallel versus perpendicular to the predominant orientation of the fibers (Table 1). Such preferential fiber reinforcement is a common practice with solid, continuous fiber-reinforced composite materials but few, if any, studies have reported successful results with highly porous materials. Despite the fact that the PGA fibers had a T_g below the testing temperature, their mechanical properties were probably less influenced by elevated temperature and water than the PLG because PGA is semi-crystalline (~50%) and the PLG is a linear, amorphous copolymer. Furthermore, the fibers may align the pore walls of the scaffold to improve the compressive properties.

When increasing amounts of PGA fibers up to 20% by weight were used to reinforce the PLG scaffolds, the compressive modulus and yield strength increased proportionally (Figure 1). This ability to control the compressive properties of the scaffolds makes fiber reinforcement a highly attractive tool for tailoring implants to specific tissue engineering applications. For example, the compressive modulus of PLG scaffolds alone (9.9 MPa) is similar to that found for bovine articular cartilage tested under similar conditions (~12 MPa) [*20*]. Furthermore, the compressive modulus of the 20% PGA/PLG scaffolds (48 MPa) is near the recommended minimum for use in trabecular bone (50 MPa) [*16*].

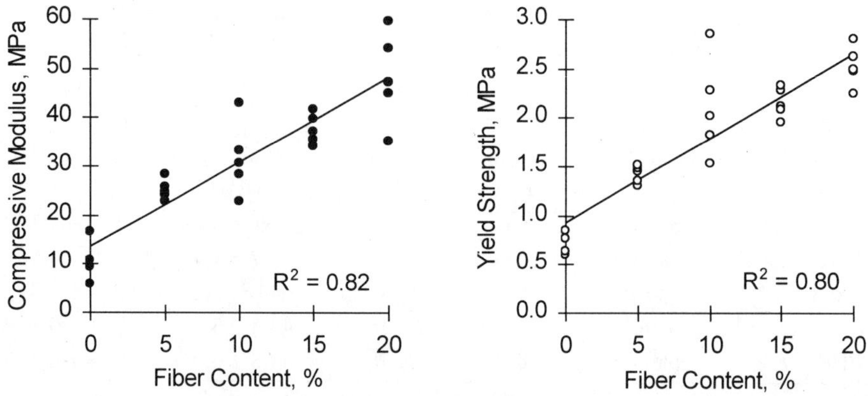

Figure 1 - *Compressive properties of fiber-reinforced PLG porous scaffolds measured in aqueous environment at 37 °C (n=5, strain rate = 0.10 min^{-1}).*

Thomson et al. have shown that porogen-leached, 85:15 D,L-PLG scaffolds with moderate porosity (47%) were effectively reinforced with short hydroxyapatite fibers (15 µm diameter, 45 µm length) up to a fiber content of 46% by weight. At 46% fiber content, the compressive yield strength reached 2.82 MPa and the compressive modulus was 82 MPa [*15*]. Although the scaffolds were tested at 37 °C, it is anticipated that the mechanical properties would decrease if tested in an aqueous environment, and therefore cannot be compared to the results from this study.

In this study, the viscoelastic properties of 10% PGA/PLG scaffolds were evaluated using compression testing over a broad range of strain rates (Figure 2). A power law relationship was found between compressive modulus (E) and strain rate (ε) over four orders of magnitude, where $E \propto \varepsilon^{0.5}$. This dependence of stiffness on strain rate can be

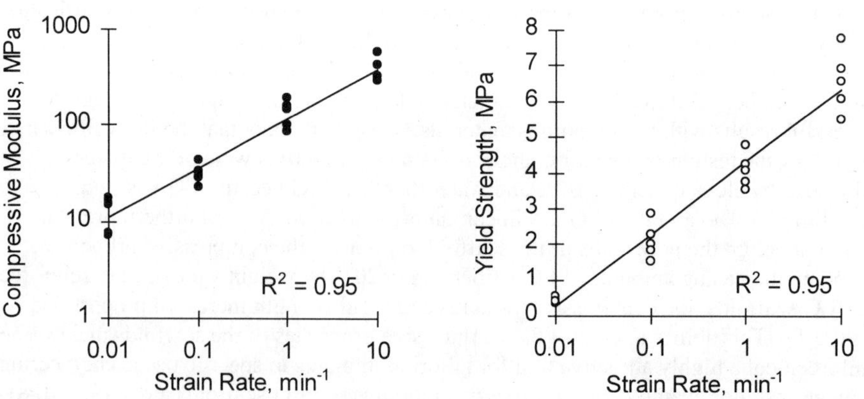

Figure 2 – *Compressive properties of 10% PGA fiber-reinforced, PLG porous scaffolds tested at four strain rates ranging four orders of magnitude (n=5, aqueous 37 °C).*

explained by two primary factors. First of all, since the scaffolds were porous and infiltrated with water, the resistance to flow of the water upon compression will likely contribute significantly to the viscous component of the viscoelastic behavior, as suggested in previous studies [*5*]. Second, most polymers have an inherent viscoelasticity, which causes their mechanical stiffness to depend highly on rate or duration of loading, as well as temperature, in well-defined ranges specific to the type of polymer [*21*]. Since the scaffolds were tested relatively close to their glass transition temperature, it is difficult to estimate the relative contributions of the two factors to the strain rate dependence. Compressive yield strength increased in a semi-logarithmic fashion with increasing strain rate (Figure 2), which is also a common trend found with viscoelastic polymers [*21*].

Upon *in vitro* degradation in PBS, the compressive modulus and yield strength of the PLG scaffolds without fiber reinforcement increased at one week, then decreased at two weeks (Figure 3), a phenomenon previously reported with 50:50 PLG [*11*], poly(phosphoester) [*6*] and poly(propylene fumarate) scaffolds [*16*]. However, results from the current study cannot be explained by cross-linking of the polymer *in vitro*, and it is highly unlikely that solvent or monomer leaching from the scaffold would be the cause, since the solvent levels were below 100 ppm and the monomer content for the raw polymers was below 0.5%. However, the use of solvents and heat drying during the manufacturing process could produce low molecular weight oligomers that would plasticize the polymer. These oligomers could then leach out during immersion *in vitro*, causing an initial increase in stiffness. An alternate reason for this behavior is the relaxation of residual stresses left over from the manufacturing process. During expansion of the polymer gel into a foam, a vacuum causes the pores to expand while

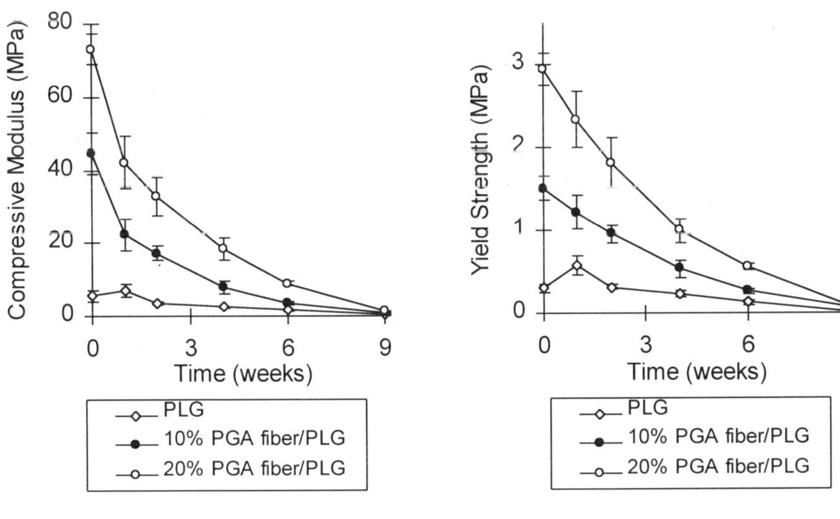

Figure 3 – *Compressive properties (mean ± standard deviation) of fiber-reinforced, PLG porous scaffolds tested after in vitro degradation in PBS (n=5, aqueous 37 °C, strain rate = 0.10 min*$^{-1}$*).*

solvent is being extracted, and there is a critical point where sufficient solvent escapes to allow the foam structure to freeze in place. Since this "freezing" occurs while the polymer molecules are being stretched under vacuum expansion, it is possible that residual contractile stresses exist after curing. A residual contractile stress would cause an apparent depression of the yield stress when tested in compression, thereby explaining why the yield strength increases when the polymer relaxes. This phenomenon was not seen with the fiber-reinforced scaffolds (Figure 3), possibly because the fibers altered the pore formation and inhibited the occurrence of residual stresses during the vacuum expansion process.

The PGA fiber-reinforced scaffolds maintained higher compressive properties throughout most of the duration of the study, but rate of loss of these properties was greater (Figure 3). In particular, the compressive modulus dropped steeply for the fiber-reinforced scaffolds at one week. It has been shown previously that PGA sutures lose approximately 15% of their tensile strength after one week of immersion in phosphate buffer (pH 7.4, 37 °C), and lose essentially all tensile strength by four weeks [*22*]. Furthermore, it has been shown that separation of the fiber-matrix interface causes early loss of mechanical properties in absorbable composites [*23-25*]. For load-bearing applications, the substantial improvement in initial strength and stiffness is desirable to provide structural support for new tissue ingrowth, and the subsequent reduction in stiffness favors gradual load transfer to the new tissue and surrounding tissues.

Conclusions

The majority of porous, absorbable scaffolds proposed for tissue engineering applications are viscoelastic, polymeric materials that are sensitive to many testing and environmental factors. Therefore, testing and reporting of the mechanical properties of these devices must be carefully planned and described in detail. Based on the results of this study, the following recommendations are made. First of all, unless it has been determined that physiological conditions do not affect the mechanical properties of the scaffold, testing should be carried out in conditions similar to the end-use environment, which will generally include an aqueous environment at 37 °C. Also, the test method or series of tests should explore the rate or time-dependence of mechanical loading to elicit the viscoelastic properties of the scaffold. Furthermore, *in vitro* or *in vivo* degradation testing should be performed to predict how the device will perform once implanted. Finally, sample dimensions, orientation of the specimen, testing method, and loading parameters must be reported for the results to be properly evaluated and for comparison with other studies.

References

[1] Freed, L. E., Grande, D. A., Lingbin, Z., Emmanual, J., Marquis, J. C., and Langer, R., "Joint Resurfacing Using Allograft Chondrocytes and Synthetic Biodegradable Polymer Scaffolds," *Journal of Biomedical Materials Research*, Vol. 28, 1994, pp. 891-899.

[2] Freed, L. E., Vunjak-Novakovic, G., Biron, R. J., Eagles, D. B., Lesnoy, D. C., Barlow, S. K., and Langer, R., "Biodegradable Polymer Scaffolds for Tissue Engineering," *Bio/Technology,* Vol. 12, 1994, pp. 689-693.

[3] Dunkelman, N., Zimber, M. P., LeBaron, R. G., Pavelec, R., Kwan, M., and Purchio, A. F., "Cartilage Production by Rabbit Articular Chondrocytes on Polyglycolic Acid Scaffolds in a Closed Bioreactor System," *Biotechnology and Bioengineering,* Vol. 46, 1995, pp. 299-305.

[4] Brittberg, M., Faxen, E., and Peterson, L., "Carbon Fiber Scaffolds in the Treatment of Early Knee Osteoarthritis: A Prospective 4-year Followup of 37 Patients," *Clinical Orthopaedics and Related Research,* Vol. 307, 1994, pp. 155-164.

[5] Lo, H., Kadiyala, S., Guggino, S. E., and Leong, K. W., "Poly(L-Lactic Acid) Foams with Cell Seeding and Controlled Release Capacity," *Journal of Biomedical Materials Research,* Vol. 30, 1996, pp. 475-484.

[6] Lo, H., Ponticiello, M. S., and Leong, K. W., "Fabrication of Controlled Release Biodegradable Foams by Phase Separation," *Tissue Engineering,* Vol. 1, No.1, 1995, pp. 15-28.

[7] Toolan, B. C., Frenkel, S. R., Pachence, J. M., Yalowitz, L., and Alexander, H., "Effects of Growth-Factor-Enhanced Culture on a Chondrocyte-Collagen Implant for Cartilage Repair," *Journal of Biomedical Materials Research,* Vol. 31, 1996, pp. 273-280.

[8] Athanasiou, K. A., Agarwal, A., and Dzida, F. J., "Comparative Study of the Intrinsic Mechanical Properties of the Human Acetabular and Femoral Head Cartilage," *Journal of Orthopaedic Research,* Vol. 12, 1994, pp. 340-349.

[9] Mikos, A. G., Sarakinos, G., Leite, S. M., Vacanti, J. P., and Langer, R., "Laminated Three-Dimensional Biodegradable Foams for Use in Tissue Engineering," *Biomaterials,* Vol. 14, No. 5, 1993, pp. 323-330.

[10] Athanasiou, K., Schmitz, J. P., and Agrawal, C. M., "The Effects of Porosity on In Vitro Degradation of Polylactic-Acid-Polyglycolic Acid Implants Used in Repair of Articular Cartilage," *Tissue Engineering,* Vol. 4, No.1, 1998, pp. 53-63.

[11] Singhal, A. R., Agrawal, C. M., and Athanasiou, K., "Salient Degradation Features of a 50:50 PLA/PGA Scaffold for Tissue Engineering," *Tissue Engineering,* Vol. 2, No.3, 1996, pp. 197-206.

[12] Zhang, R. and Ma, P. X., "Poly(α-Hydroxyl Acids)/Hydroxyapatite Porous Composites for Bone-Tissue Engineering. I. Preparation and Morphology," *Journal of Biomedical Materials Research,* Vol. 44, No.4, 1999, pp. 446-455.

[13] DeGroot, J. H., Nijenhuis, A. J., Bruin, P., Pennings, A. J., Veth, R. P. H., Klompmaker, J., and Jansen, H. W. B., "Use of Porous Biodegradable Polymer

Implants in Meniscus Reconstruction. 1) Preparation of Porous Biodegradable Polyurethanes for the Reconstruction of Meniscus Lesions," *Colloid & Polymer Science,* Vol. 268, 1990, pp. 1073-1081.

[14] Thomson, R. C., Yaszemski, M. J., Powers, J. M., and Mikos, A. G., "Fabrication of Biodegradable Polymer Scaffolds to Engineer Trabecular Bone," *Journal of Biomaterial Science, Polymer Edition,* Vol. 7, No.1, 1995, pp. 23-38.

[15] Thomson, R. C., Yaszemski, M. J., Powers, J. M., and Mikos, A. G., "Hydroxyapatite Fiber Reinforced Poly(α-hydroxy ester) Foams for Bone Regeneration," *Biomaterials,* Vol. 19, 1998, pp. 1935-1943.

[16] Peter, S. J., Nolley, J. A., Widmer, M. S., Merwin, J. E., Yaszemski, M. j., Yasko, A. W., Engel, P. S., and Mikos, A. G., "*In Vitro* Degradation of a Poly(Propylene Fumarate)/β-Tricalcium Phosphate Composite Orthopaedic Scaffold," *Tissue Engineering,* Vol. 3, No.2, 1997, pp. 207-215.

[17] Slivka, M. A., Leatherbury, N. C., Kieswetter, K., and Niederauer, G. G., "Resorbable Scaffolds Tailored for Articular Cartilage Repair using Fiber Reinforcement," *Transactions of the Society for Biomaterials*, Society for Biomaterials, Providence, RI, 1999, p. 525.

[18] Niederauer, G. G., Slivka, M. A., Leatherbury, N. C., Korvick, D. L., and Kieswetter, K., "Multiphase Implants with Varying Stiffness Affect Osteochondral Cartilage Repair," *Transactions of the Society for Biomaterials*, Society for Biomaterials, Providence, RI, 1999, p. 261.

[19] Thompson, D. E., Agrawal, C. M., and Athanasiou, K., "The Effects of Dynamic Compressive Loading on Biodegradable Implants of 50-50% Polylactic Acid-Polyglycolic Acid," *Tissue Engineering,* Vol. 2, No.1, 1996, pp. 61-73.

[20] Oloyede, A., Flachsmann, R., and Broom, N. D., "The Dramatic Influence of Loading Velocity on the Compressive Response of Articular Cartilage," *Connective Tissue Research,* Vol. 27, 1992, pp. 211-224.

[21] Rodriguez, F., "Mechanical Properties at Small Deformations," *Principles of Polymer Systems*, Hemisphere Publishing, New York, 1989, pp. 229-261.

[22] Chu, C. C., "The In Vitro Degradation of Polyglycolic Acid Sutures - Effect of pH," *Journal of Biomedical Materials Research,* Vol. 15, 1981, pp. 795-804.

[23] Slivka, M. A., Chu, C. C., and Adisaputro, I. A., "Fiber-Matrix Interface Studies on Bioabsorbable Composite Materials for Internal Fixation of Bone Fractures. I. Raw Material Evaluation and Measurement of Fiber-Matrix Interfacial Adhesion," *Journal of Biomedical Materials Research,* Vol. 36, No.4, 1997, pp. 469-477.

[24] Slivka, M. A. and Chu, C. C., "Fiber-Matrix Interface Studies on Bioabsorbable Composite Materials for Internal Fixation of Bone Fractures. II. A New Method Using Laser Scanning Confocal Microscopy," *Journal of Biomedical Materials Research,* Vol. 37, No.3, 1997, pp. 353-362.

[25] Zimmerman, M. C., Alexander, H., Parsons, J. R., and Bajpai, P. K., "The Design and Analysis of a Laminated Partially Degradable Composite Bone Plate for Fracture Fixation," *Journal of Biomedical Materials Research: Applied Biomaterials,* Vol. 21, No.A3, 1987, pp. 345-361.

Dietmar W. Hutmacher,[1] Axel Kirsch,[2] Karl L. Ackermann,[2] Markus B. Hürzeler[3]

Clinical Evaluation of a Bioresorbable Membrane for Hard Tissue Regeneration

---

Reference: Hutmacher, D. W., Kirsch, A., Ackermann, K. L., and Hürzeler, M. B., "**Clinical Evaluation of a Bioresorbable Membrane for Hard Tissue Regeneration,**" *Synthetic Bioabsorbable Polymers for Implants, STP 1396,* C. M. Agrawal, J. E. Parr and S. T. Lin, Eds., American Society for Testing and Materials, West Conshohocken, PA, 2000.

Abstract: In the field of guided bone regeneration, biomedical engineering has been applied, more or less successfully, to the development of biodegradable and bioresorbable membranes whose chemical, physical, or mechanical properties, structure, or form permits active tissue integration of desirable cell types and tissue components. The employment of synthetic and naturally occurring polymers as well as sophisticated manufacturing technologies allow the design and fabrication of matrix configurations, so that the biophysical limitations for guided bone regeneration can be satisfied. The configuration of such a hybrid matrix can also be manipulated to vary the surface area available for cell attachment, as well as to optimize the exposure of the attached cells to nutrients. A bioresorbable membrane made of synthetic and natural polymers has been developed and manufactured. This innovative device concept has been applied as guided bone regeneration (GBR) membrane.

Keywords: guided bone regeneration, biodegradable and bioresorbable membranes

Introduction

Over the last two decades, experimental and clinical studies on periodontal wound healing have resulted in the development of a regenerative treatment modality called

---

[1]Laboratory for Biomedical Engineering /Department of Orthopedic Surgery, National University of Singapore, 10 Kent Ridge Crescent, Singapore 119260
[2] Private Practice, Stuttgart-Filderstadt, Germany
[3] Department of Restorative Dentistry and Periodontology, Albert Ludwigs University Freiburg, Germany

community has gained extensive experience in implementing the GBR-technique in its treatment regimes. The objective of guided bone regeneration is to promote bone formation in osseous deformities, either before or in conjunction with endosseous implant placement. Osseous defects consist mainly of extraction sites, dehiscence, and/or fenestration's as well as localized ridge deformities. Furthermore, bone defect geometry may either provide natural spacemaking or be non-spacemaking. Presently, the GBR technique is supported by a significant number of experimental and clinical studies, randomized and non-randomized [*1-16*]. The clinical goal of GBR is to create a suitable environment in which the natural biological potential for functional regeneration can be maximized [*2-4,6,7,15,17-20*].

It has become clear that tissue separation is only one of many interacting factors that influence the predictability and success of GBR treatment concepts. Important factors involved in the creation of a suitable environment for GBR procedures include: biomechanical stability of the resolving wound complex, prevention of acute inflammation resulting from salvia bacterial infection, isolation of the regenerative space from undesirable competing tissue types, and creation and maintenance of a blood clot filled space. While certainly not the only critical component to successful GBR-treatment, the material properties and membrane design employed in the therapy can significantly influence all of the above-mentioned factors.

Historically, designers of GTR membranes have ´ borrowed ´ polymeric materials as well as manufacturing technologies originally developed for other bioresorbable devices, e.g., sutures, dressings, screws, and plates. Basic biomedical engineering principles have been applied to the design and fabrication of GTR devices more or less successfully - resulting in biodegradable and bioresorbable membranes whose chemical, physical, or mechanical properties, structure, or form may permit passive and non-inductive tissue integration of desirable cell types and tissue components. There appears to be a consensus that biodegradable and bioresorbable membranes designed for GTR procedures have to retain their physical barrier function for at least 4 to 6 weeks and membranes and devices for GBR treatment concepts for 6 to 9 months [*6-8,11*]. Unfortunately at present, there is no bioresorbable membrane uniquely designed for GBR treatment concepts commercially available.

From a clinical point of view, cell occlusive devices specifically designed for GBR treatment regimes have to be developed. In addition, special processing and manufacturing techniques have to be evaluated to incorporate drugs and/or biological agents without inactivation, into a bioresorbable membrane matrix to enhance the clinical predictability of the treatment concepts practicing guided bone regeneration techniques.

General Requirements for a Bioresorbable Membrane

The functional requirements for all physical barrier devices used in GBR procedures are the same, regardless of whether they are non-resorbable, biodegradable, or bioresorbable. However, the material properties and characteristics, e.g., chemical, biochemical and physical, have to be different, to allow for the performance of the intended function. Hardwick [*18,19*] and Scantlebury [*20*] suggest that five design criteria may be applied to the selection of appropriate materials and designs for specific GBR applications: biocompatibility, cell-occlusivity, spacemaking, tissue integration, and clinical applicability. These criteria determine the efficacy of non-resorbable, bioresorbable and biodegradable membranes. However, the chemical, physical, and biochemical properties to fulfill these criteria differ from one biomaterial to the other.

To date, there is no scientific proof for the micro- and macrostructure for the first choice of bioresorbable membranes used for GBR treatment regimes. Dense, fully occlusive devices offer the advantage of having a small surface area and, hence, a low degradation and resorption rate per volume. Microporous devices, which allow for fluid and oxygen exchange, provide a considerably greater surface area per volume and thereby may be subject to a much faster degradation and resorption. Experimental studies on the importance of membrane permeability suggest that the exchange of fluids is not necessary for the supply of the newly forming bone under the membrane. Schmid et al [*21*] placed titanium test cylinders of 0.05 cm^3 volume onto the foreheads of rabbits. Different structured e-PTFE membranes either covered the cylinders, or they were sealed off by cast titanium as a control. After eight months, for all animals and all sites, equal amounts of new cancellous bone formation were observed histologically within both test and control cylinders. Differences in membrane permeability did not appear to influence the bone regeneration process. The author concludes that membrane permeability is not required for new bone formation when applying the GBR methodology. However, it is known that bone can survive on diffusion across a distance of approximately 5 mm from the underlying host bone [*6*]. The nutrient supply and waste disposal of the newly forming bone may thus be well accomplished, solely by the underlying bone in GBR in small- and medium-volume bone defects. However, it seems questionable whether or not an exchange of oxygen and body fluids through membrane porosities is important in large volume defects.

The ability to create and maintain a given space with desired geometry adjacent to the parent bone surface is a critical requirement for successful GBR applications. The spacemaking or resistance-to-collapse properties of a membrane designed for GBR are important considerations in the choice of an appropriate device material. Schliephake et al [*22-24*] have explored the potential for bioresorbable, pre-formed, or in situ shapeable devices in large defect models or in situations where adjacent anatomy is not conducive to membrane support. With additional stiffness pre-forming the membrane, or designing the device to be shapeable, it is necessary to allow close adaptation of the membrane to the surfaces of the bone peripheral to the defect.

The Design Concept

The tissue engineered cell occlusive device of our interdisciplinary research group was made in a sandwich design: two collagen membranes with a synthetic polymer component in between (Figure 1a/b). The synthetic polymer component can be designed and manufactured non-porous, like a film/sheet, or porous like a membrane. The synthetic film/membrane thickness can be varied between 200 μm and 500 μm. The aliphatic polyester layer provide the physical barrier device the following physical properties: cell occlusivity, a physical barrier function for 6 to 9 months (Figure 2), and the capability to maintain a given space under biomechanical soft tissue load.

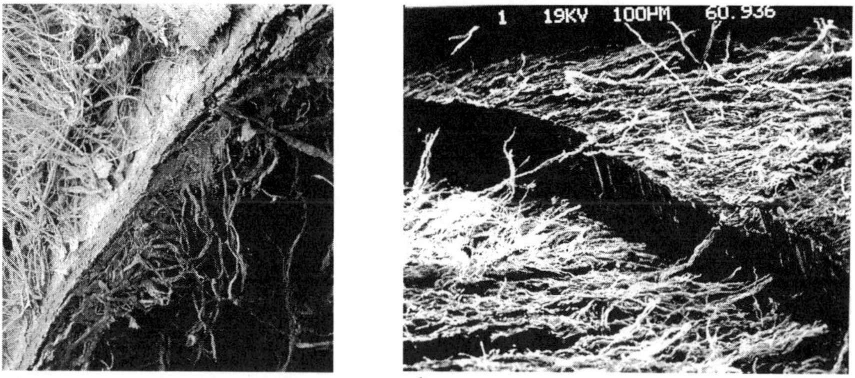

a b

Figure 1a/b - *Cross section of freeze fractured surfaces of a composite membrane with a non porous poly (L-lactide-co-D,L-lactide) 70/30 layer. The collagen fiber bundles are closely bonded on the synthetic polymer surface*

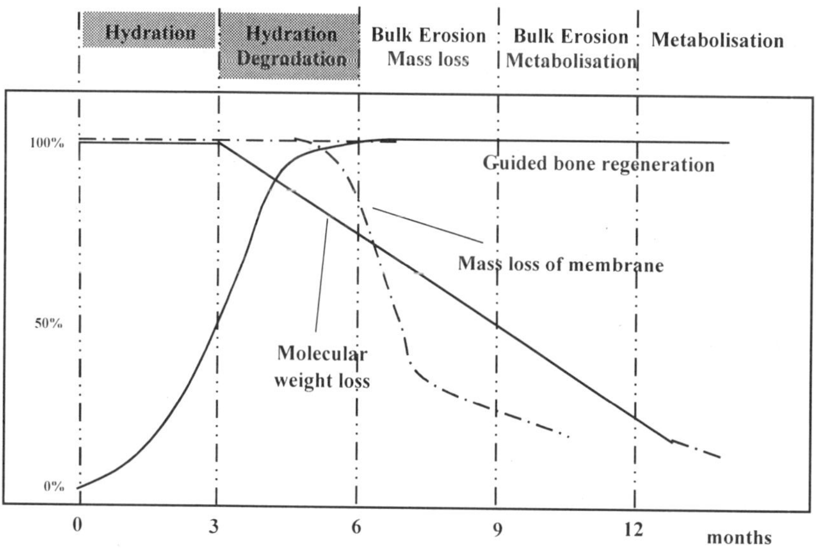

Figure 2 - *Graphical illustration of the ideal degradation and resorption kinetics for a physical barrier membrane specifically designed for guided bone regeneration*

Poly (α-hydroxy acids) can be easily shaped if the macromolecules are heated past their glass transition temperature (T_g). The T_gs for polylactides and polyglycolides, which are relatively stiff and brittle at room temperature, range from 45 to 60^0 C depending on the polymer composition. Hence, the hybrid membrane becomes more flexible in situ due to the body temperature of 37 ^{0} C. Pre-forming of the device in regard to a specific bone defect geometry is also possible.

The Rationale of Collagen in the Design Concept

Of the naturally occurring polymers used in surgery, collagen is by far the most intensely studied biomaterials. Collagens have been used as suture material for over a century [*25*]. In general, it is derived from submucosa of bovine or bovine intestine. In an effort to reduce the antigenic response of processed collagen-based materials, methods of dissociation, purification, and reconstitution of collagen have been developed [*26-28*]. The source of such collagen is usually animal tendon or hide. The reconstitution process yields a pure, less antigenic collagen.

Due to the superior tissue-integration function in as compared by synthetic polymers, collagen has been a topic of increasing interest for the design and processing of membranes for GBR procedures as well as matrix material for bone morphogenetic proteins. However, the use of a pure collagen membrane for GBR procedures is very limited, firstly, due to its lack of spacemaking properties, and secondly, due to inefficient degradation kinetics [*29-31*].

The strong clinical benefits of bioresorbable devices that have the capacity to integrate with the surrounding soft and hard tissue results in a more mechanically stable and therefore predictable wound-healing environment. Since collagen membranes do not have spacemaking properties, they need a second biodegradable or bioresorbable material to fulfill this criteria, e.g., a poly (α-hydroxy acid) component as demonstrated in our tissue engineered cell occlusive device.

The Role of a Inorganic Filler in the Design Concept

The incorporation of a ceramic bone substitute - e.g. tricalciumphosphate or hydroxyapatite - in the bioresorbable synthetic polymer produces a hybrid/composite material (Figure 3), which improves the mechanical properties and supports triggering of the desired degradation and resorption kinetics [*32*]. The membrane compression molded of a pure aliphatic polyester has a rather hydrophobic surface. A hydrophilic surface would improve biocompatibility and subsequently the hard tissue generation in a way that ceramic particles, which are embedded into the polymer matrix, allow for an extended surface binding of serum proteins. In addition, the basic resorption products of the inorganic material would buffer the acidic resorption by-products of the aliphatic polyester and may thereby help to avoid the formation of an unfavorable environment for the cells due to a decreased pH [*32*]. However, a disadvantage from a clinical application point of view arises because the device becomes very stiff and is difficult to surgically place it on the host bone a geometrical complex defect.

The Applied Manufacturing Technology

The gradual shift from non-resorbable membranes to bioresorbable membranes represents one of the most significant trends in modern GBR treatment regimes. Unfortunately, investigators seeking advanced GBR devices are severely limited not only in candidate polymeric biomaterials, but also by sophisticated manufacturing and processing technologies. This is evident from the relatively small number of different processing and design concepts described in the scientific GTR/GBR literature. Two processing technologies have been studied to manufacture prototypes of the new device, namely compression molding and the supercritical fluid-gassing process.

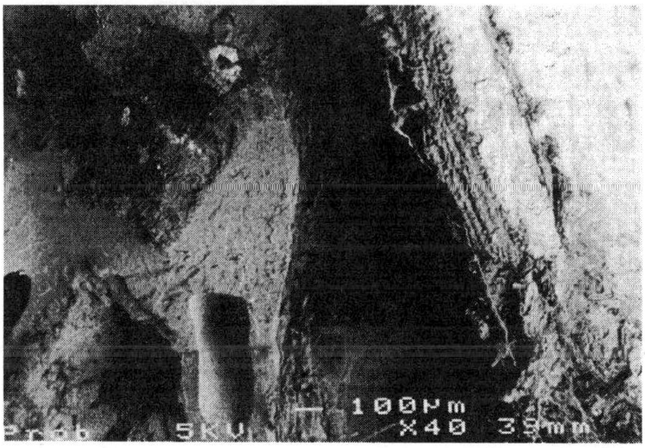

Figure 3 - *SEM picture of a freeze fractured surface of a composite-membrane with a middle layer composed of poly (L-lactide-co-D,L-lactide) and coral hydroxyapatite particles (300-500 μm) in a 80/ 20 weight ratio.*

Compression Molding

Sheets of a regular thickness of (0.2+0,08 mm and 0.4 + 0,1 mm) were processed on a Dr. Collin Labaratory Four Column Press ((Dr. Collin GmbH, Ebersberg Germany). Poly (lactide-co-D,L-lactide) 70/30 (Boehringer Ingelheim, Ingelheim Germany) in separate amounts of 12.9 g and 25.8 were placed on a 4mm thick steel plate covered with a polytetrafluoethylene release film (Airtech International, Carson, CA) and placed on the lower press platen. A 0.2 mm or 0.4 mm thick steel frame and a 4mm thick steel plate, also covered with a polytetrafluorethylene release film, were added to the top. The press platens were then heated to a temperature of 204 $^{\circ}$C and maintained without pressure for 20 minutes. A force ramp of 5 to10 to 20 to 40 bar was applied over a period of 15 minutes. Then the platens were quick quenched to room temperature under a pressure of 40 bar. The press was released and the 0.2 mm or 0,4 mm poly (lactide-co-D,L-lactide) 70/30 films were removed.

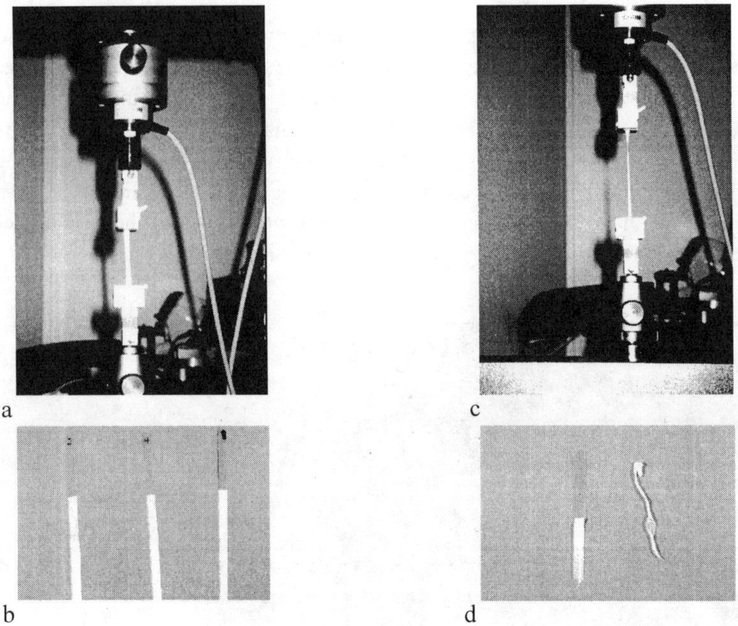

Figure 4 a-d - *The bonding strength of bi-layered composite specimens (110x5 mm) has been studied using a delamination test on a mechanical tester (Karl Franck GmbH, Mutterstadt, Germany). As shown in Figure 3d the collagen and poly (lactide-co-D,L-lactide) 70/30 layers did not delaminate. The collagen membrane itself did fail, indicating that the wet bonding strength between the thermally fused synthetic and natural polymer is sufficient for clinical application.*

The sandwich like (Figure 1a/b) and bi-layered constructs (Figure 4b/d) were fabricated using an ultra short heat pressing cycle. For the clinical study 200 and 400 μm thick poly (lactide-co-D,L-lactide) 70/30 sheets were thermally fused with two 400 μm thick collagen sheets (clinical case 1 and 2). The type I/III collagen membranes (Biogide, Geistlich Biomaterials, Wollhusen, Switzerland) were fabricated from the soft tissue of piglets. The overall thickness of the composite device measured 500 μm after the heat pressing. A delamination test (ASTM D 5824-98) was performed to evaluate the bonding between the synthetic and natural polymers under three different conditions (Figure 4a/c). In group I the temperature was 100 °C and a pressure of 5 bar was applied for 10 seconds, whereas in group II at the same temperature and pressure the fusion cycle was 20 seconds. Specimens of group III were treated for 10 seconds at a temperature of 120 °C and a pressure of 5 bar. A collagen assay was performed and revealed that the type I and III collagen had not degraded during the short term thermal treatment. The test bi-layered specimen (Figure 4b,d) were soaked in a sterile saline solution at a temperature of 37 °C for 15 minutes. The average bond strength of the tested specimens of group I was 6,7 N, group II 6.9 N, and group III 7.3 N.

Supercritical Fluid-Gassing Technology

The supercritical fluid-gassing process has been known for many years in the non-medical polymer industry [*33*] as well as in the pharmaceutical community [*34*]. This technology is used to produce foams and other highly porous products. The polymers, which can be applied by this technology, have to be mainly amorphous. The polymer granules are plasticized due to the employment of a gas such as nitrogen or carbon dioxide at high pressure. The diffusion and dissolution of the gas into the polymer matrix results in a reduction of the viscosity, which allows the processing of the amorphous bioresorbable polyesters in a temperature range of 30 to 40 °C.

The so-called `low process temperature technology` constitutes a new manufacturing process within the biomaterial and biomedical research society - opening up new potential applications, particularly in the development of bioresorbable devices [*35*]. The supercritical fluid-gassing technology allows the incorporation of heat sensitive pharmaceuticals and biological agents. Conventional mold technology permits the development of made-to-measure bioresorbable carrier systems with a drug delivery function for the individual patient.

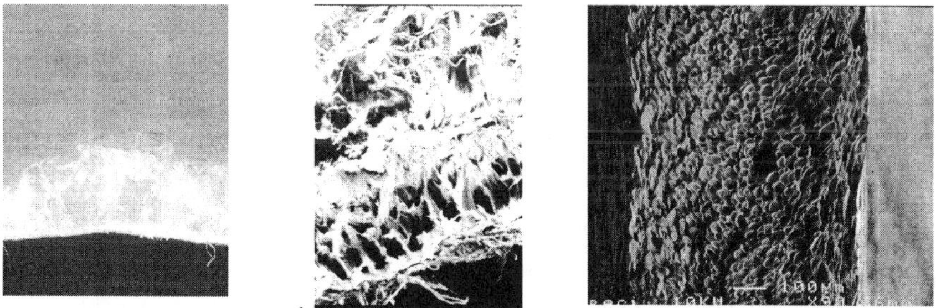

a b c

Figure 5a-c - The composite membrane fabricated by applying the super-critical fluid gassing technology (a). The synthetic polymer matrix has a highly porous structure and exhibited a good bonding to the collagen sheets (b,c).

Supercritical-fluid gassing technology was applied for fabricating the composite membranes (Figure 5a-c). From the experimental data, the limitations of supercritical-gassing technology can be reported [*36*]: I. the poly (lactide-co-D,L-lactide) 70/30 layer cannot be fabricated thinner than 400 μm, II. only 20% to 30% of the microcellular structure was interconnected, III. Lyophilization of the polymer granules in combination with the water-based growth factor solution prevents the gas from diffusing into the macromolecular polymer structure, IV. Mixing of the polymer granules with a lyophilized growth factor results in a non-homogenous distribution (Figure 6), V. Skinning effect on the outer matrix surface. Predictably, none of the composite membranes processed by the supercritical-fluid gassing technology have been applied clinically, yet.

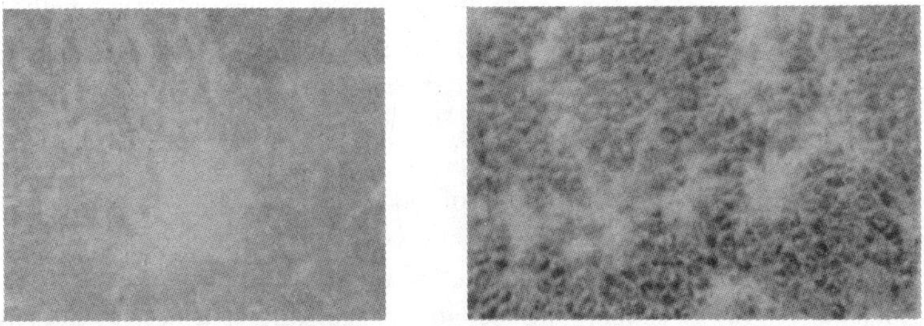

a b

Figure 6a/b *Light microscopical picture of a porous poly (D,L-lactide) membrane. The basic fibroblast growth factor (bFGF) (Merck, Darmstadt, Germany) have been incorporated by the supercritical foaming technology. The inhomogeneous distribution of the lyophilized bFGF in the microcellular architecture and the low interconnectivity of the pores is visible in the higher magnification (Figure 6b).*

Clinical Evaluation

The purpose of the preliminary clinical evaluation was to study the ability of a tissue engineered cell occlusive device to function as a physical barrier without a clinically detectable foreign body reaction. Between December 1, 1995 and September 31, 1997 seven patients - scheduled for prosthetic implant treatment presented with inadequate bone volume for implant placement – have been included in the clinical evaluation of the new composite membrane in bone graft donor sites.

Clinical and radiographic examinations were performed to evaluate the bone graft donor sites. The choice of donor site, either symphysis or ramus, was determined preoperatively based on defect morphology and recipient site location. A panoramic radiograph was used to map the course of the inferior alveolar canal. Lateral cephalometric, posterior-anterior projections, and periapical radiographs were also used when necessary to assess the donor sites. The recipient site had completely healed prior to graft surgery. Tooth extractions were completed at least 8 weeks before grafting.

The patient group from a private practice comprised 5 women (71,4%) and two men (28,6%). The mean age of the patients at the time of surgery was 56,4 years. The mandibular symphysis (Figure 7a/b) was used as a donor site in four, the ramus in one, and dental implant dehiscence (Figure 8a/b) in two cases. Patients were not accepted for endosseous implant surgery if they did not fulfill the general requirements for surgery. Postoperative observation ranged from 12 to 32 months. All patients experienced uneventful healing during this time period. Slight inflammation was observed at all sites for the first 2 weeks of healing. This was especially apparent at the wound margins. In no patient was a dehiscence or suppuration observed throughout the healing period. One patient experienced the incidence of temporary mental nerve paresthesia in symphysis graft patients. The ramus graft patient noted no soft tissue sensory deficits. None of the symphysis graft patients described altered sensation of the incisor teeth.

From two patients, a trephine drill biopsy was be obtained 12 and 15 months postoperatively (Figure 7c-e). The histological sections taken from the augmented area after showed cellular woven bone and Bio-Oss particles with an apposition of osteoid in which was direct contact. The physical barrier device itself was absent, indicating complete degradation of the device. However, small polymer particles could be detected meaning that the resorption and metabolization process of the PLLA/PDLA 70/30 layer was in his final stage. Fibrous connective tissue was present with fibroblasts. The graft–connective tissue interface showed no inflammatory infiltrate. Qualitative evaluation of the specimens revealed a slight invasion of the fibrous connective tissue into the graft material at a microscopic level. Fragments of vital and non-vital bone surrounded by connective tissue were seen at the graft surface. Small blood vessels were also evident. Although few in number, vital bone fragment were seen with lining cells. Small deposits of osteoid were present, and giant cells were sparse (Figure 7e).

Case 1

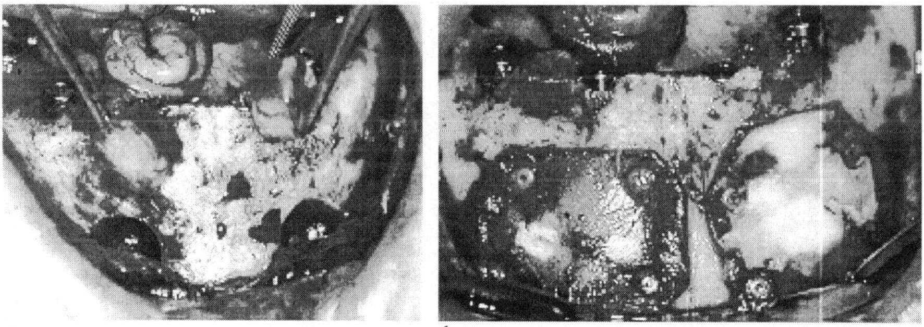

a b

Figure 7a/b - *Symphysis Donor Site: Fixation and stabilization of two composite membranes - a physiological requirement in protecting the blood clot and maintaining close adaptation of the membrane to the bone surface during the entire bone regeneration period – was achieved by applying bioresorbable minipins.*

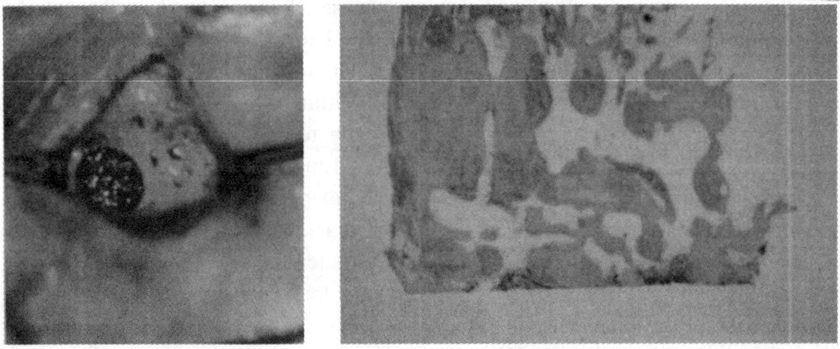

c d

Figure 7c/d - *Clinical view on the biopsy site (Figure 7c). A 3 mm-diameter trephine drill was used to drill the graft site to prepare a core graft material at least 6 mm in length. This technique allowed a histologic view of the osseous graft soft tissue interface with minimal distortion. Photomicrograph of a gross specimen obtained from trephine drill biopsy, 12 months postoperatively (Figure 7d). The application of the composite membrane resulted in new bone formation and bone apposition to the BioOss granules. The physical barrier device itself was absent, indicating complete degradation of the tissue engineered cell occlusive device. (original magnification x 8; toluidine blue stain).*

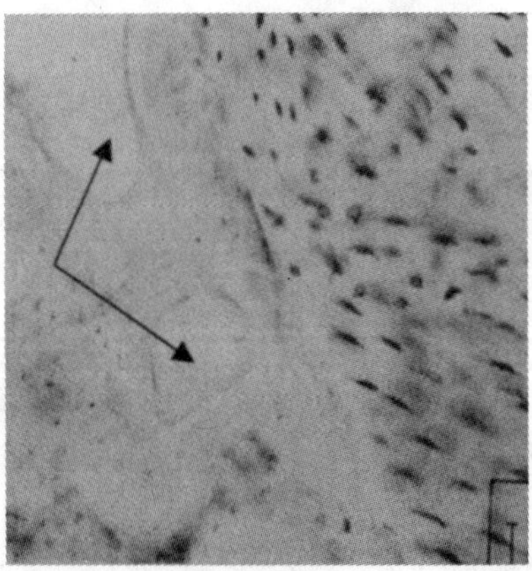

Figure 7e - *High magnification photomicrograph shows fibrous connective tissue with fibroblasts. The graft–connective tissue interface reveals no inflammatory infiltrate. Fragments of vital and non-vital bone surrounded by connective tissue were seen at the graft surface. Low molecular weight particles (arrows) can be detected microscopically specifying that the resorption and metabolization process of the PLLA/PDLA 70/30 layer is in its final stage (original magnification x 40; toluidine blue stain).*

Case 2

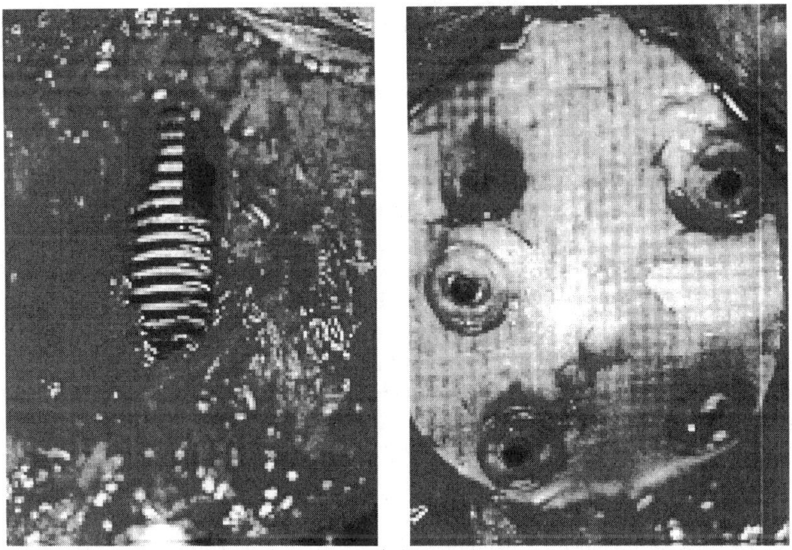

a b

Figure 8 a/b - *Placement of the composite device construct over the three dimensional bone defect after dental implant placement. Fixation and stabilization of the composite membranes - a physiological requirement in protecting the blood clot and maintaining close adaptation of the multi-layered construct to the bone surface during the entire bone regeneration period – was achieved by applying five bioresorbable minipins.*

Discussion

The successful use of a e-PTFE membrane in periodontology established the basis for the technique of guided bone regeneration in implant dentistry [1-4]. Attempts to solve initial problems with membrane collapses have been tried using membrane-supporting screws [37-39]. Another treatment option is to fill the space underneath the membrane with a autogenous bone graft or bone substitutes, such as hydroxyapatite and tricalciumphosphate to maintain the contour [40]. But neither measure solved the problem of the reduced membrane stiffness. As a consequence, titanium-reinforced e-PTFE membranes are now available [41-43].

Another drawback of e-PTFE membranes is the risk of infection after wound dehiscence. Bacterial contamination of the exposed membrane cannot be avoided, even when the patient is taking antibiotics or using antiseptic mouth rinses. If an exposed e-PTFE membrane is not removed in time, a wound infection eventually occurs [44].

Hence, the clinical result will be compromised because the hard tissue regeneration process is disturbed [45].

The advantage of biodegradable and bioresorbable physical barriers for GBR treatment concepts is the obviation of the surgical intervention after the device has fulfilled its mission. Hence, another treatment option is to utilize a bi-layered collagen membrane specifically developed for GBR [40,46]. Due to poor mechanical properties, this type of physical barrier membrane bears the risk of collapsing. Hence, a defect filler is needed to prevent the downfall. In contrast the cell occlusive device described in this paper, while almost as stiff as a titanium mesh, can be easily trimmed and molded to the desired morphology in a three dimensional bone architecture. The added stiffness is an advantage because it provides greater resistance to deformation during healing than does a conventional e-PTFE or collagen membrane. However, in a large three dimensional bone defect, pre-formed composite devices have to be used. Our interdisciplinary research team has been recently working on such a design concept [47].

The degradation, resorption and metabolization process will, by definition, have associated with it some inflammatory cellular response in the surrounding tissue, regardless of whether the material is broken down by hydrolysis or through enzymatic mechanisms. This inflammatory response should be minimal and reversible, and it must not be detrimental to the conditions of bone regeneration. The process should be controlled so that the physical properties of the material is maintained during the initial healing period and the function for hard tissue guidance is maintained for a sufficient length of time. The multi-layered device made of two collagen membranes and a synthetic copolymer sheet appear to meet these criteria.

Conclusion

In conclusion, the supercritical fluid-gassing technology, as well as compression molding, has been applied to process a bioresorbable device for GBR procedures whose design concept has been described in this paper. Although, the first clinical application of the new physical barrier specifically designed for GBR procedures is indeed promising, a number of controlled animal and clinical studies are needed before such a device developed from a tissue engineering point of view can be considered clinically established. Today, different types and designs of the so-called " composite membrane "- with and without biological agents such as growth factors and peptides - are being investigated in several experimental and clinical studies.

Acknowledgement

The authors would like to thank Oliver Pfannschmidt of the IKV Aachen for the support of fabricating the composite membranes by the super-critical fluid technology, Manoja Ranawake for critical reading of the manuscript, and the Dr.Collin GmbH for use of the Technikum.

References

[1] Mellonig J.T., Nevins M., Guided bone regeneration of bone defects associated with implants: An evidence-based outcome assessment. J Periodontics Restorative Dentistry 1995; Vol.15:169-184.

[2] Buser, D., Dula, K., Hirt, H.P., Berthold, H., "Localized ridge augmentation using guided bone regeneration", Buser, D., Dahlin, C., Schenk, K.R. (eds.), Guided bone regeneration in implant dentistry, Quintessence, 1994, pp 189-234.

[3] Linde A, Alberius P, Dahlin C, Bjurstam K, Sundin Y. Osteopromotion. A soft tissueexclusion principle using a membrane for bone healing and bone neogenesis. J Periodont 1993; 64:1116-1128

[4] Dahlin C, Andersson L, Linde A. Bone augmentation at fenestrated implants by an osteopromotive membrane technique. A controlled clinical study. Clin Ora Impl Res 1991; 2:159-165

[5] Zellin G, Gritli-Linde A, Linde A. Healing of mandibular defects with different biodegradable and non-degradable membranes: an experimental study in rats. Biomaterials 1995; 16:601-609

[6] Schenk R.K, Buser D, Hardwick WR, Dahlin C. Healing pattern of bone regeneration in membrane-protected defects. Int J Oral Maxillofac Implants 1994; 9:13-29

[7] Buser D., Schenk RK. Standortbestimmung der membrangeschuetzten Knochen-regeneration in der oralen Implantologie. Teil 1 : Wissenschaftliche Grundlagen. Implantologie 1995, 3:209-226

[8] Buser D, Schenk R.K., Standortbestimmung der membrangeschuetzten Knochen-regeneration in der oralen Implantologie. Teil 2: Chirurgische Technik, Implantologie 1995, 4:301-312

[9] Gottlw J., Guided tissue regeneration using bioresorbable and non-resorbable devices: Initial healing and long-term results. J Peridontol 1993; 64,11:1157-1165.

[10] Gottlow J., Laurell L., Rylander H., Lundgren D, Rudolfsson I, Nyman S: Treatment of infrabony defects in monkeys with bioresorbable and non-resorbable guided tissue regeneration devices. J Dent Res 1993; 72 (special issue):824.

[11] Kirsch A, Ackermann K L, Hürzeler M B, Dürr W, Hutmacher D. Gesteuerte Knochenregeneration - 5 Jahre klinische Erfahrung mit der Applikation von Titanmembrannaegeln zur Fixation von nicht-resorbierbaren Membranen. Implantologie 1996, 4: 289-297

[12] Hürzeler MB, Weng D, Hutmacher D. Knochenregneration um Implantate - eine klinische Studie mit einer neuen resorbierbaren Membran. Deutsche Zahnaerztliche Zeitschrift 1996, 51 Jahrgang, Vol 5: 1-7

[13] Hutmacher D, Kirsch A, Ackermann KL, Hürzeler MB. Entwicklung eines bioresorbierbaren Membranfixationsystems. Z Zahnärztl Implantol 1996, 12:141-147

[14] Jovanovic SA, Buser D. Guided bone regeneration in dehiscence defects and delayed extraction sockets. in: Guided bone regeneration in implant dentistry (eds.): Buser D, Dahlin C, Schenk RK, 1994) p 155-188

[15] Dahlin, C.: Scientific background of guided bone regeneration. In: Buser, D., Dahlin, C., Schenk, K.R. (eds.): Guided bone regeneration in implant dentistry. Quintessence, Chicago 1994, p.31.

[16] Lang, N.P., Haemmerle, C.F., Braegger, U., Lehmann, B., Nyman, S.: Guided tissue regeneration in jawbone defects prior to implant placement. Clin Oral Implant Res 5, 92 (1994).

[17] Buser D., Dula K, Hirt HP, Schenk R. Lateral Ridge Augmentation Using Autografts and Barrier Membranes: A Clinical Study With 40 partially Edentulous patients. J Oral Maxillofac Surg 54: 420-432, 1996

[18] Hardwick R, Scantlebury V T, Sanchez R, Whitely N, Ambruster J: Membrane design criteria for guided bone regeneration of the alveolar ridge. Guided bone regeneration in implant dentistry. edited by Buser D, Dahlin C, Schenk K R; 101-136.

[19] Hardwick R, Hayes KB, Flynn C: Devices for dentoalveolar regeneration: An up-to-dateliterature review. J Peridontol 1995; 66,6:495-505

[20] Scantlebury V T: 1982-1992: A decade of technology development for guided tissue regeneration. J Peridontol 1993; 64,11:1129-1137.

[21] Schmid J, Haemmerle F H C, Olah J A, Lang P N: Membrane permeability is unnecessary for guided regeneration of new bone. An experimental study in the rabbit. Clin Oral Im Res 1994 ; 3:125-130

[22] Schliephake H, Neukam W F, Hutmacher D, Becker J: Enhancement of bone ingrowth into a porous hydroxyapatite-matrix using a resorbable polylactic membrane. J Oral Maxillofac Surg 1994; 52:57-63.

[23] Schliephake H, Neukam W F, Hutmacher D, Whstenfeld H: Experimental transplantation of HA-bone composite grafts. J Oral Maxillofac Surg 1994; 53:46-51

[24] Schliephake H, Neukam W F, Hutmacher D, Becker J: The use of a basic fibroblast growth factor (bFGF) for enhancement of bone ingrowth into pyrolized bovine bone. Int J Oral Maxillofac Surg 1994; 52:57-63

[25] Hutmacher D, Hürzeler M, Schliephake H. A review of material properties of biodegradable and bioresorbable polymers and devices for GTR and GBR applications. Int J Oral Maxillofac Implants 1996; 11:667-678

[26] Burgeson R, Morris N P. The collagen family of proteins. Uitto J, Perejda A J, eds. Connective tissue disease, New York, Marcell DekkerInc., 1987:23-27

[27] Salthouse T M. Cellular enzyme activity at the polymer-tissue interface: A review. J Biomed Mater Res 1986; 10:197

[28] Huang C, Yannas I V. Mechanical studies of enzymatic degradation of insoluble collagen fibres. J Biomed Mater Res 1977; 8:137.

[29] Huerzeler, M.B., Kohal, R.J., Naghsbandi, J., Mota, L.F., Conradt, J., Hutmacher, D., Caffesse, R.G. Evaluation of a new bioresorbable barrier to facilitate bone regeneration around exposed implant threads. An experimental study in the monkey. Int J Oral Maxillofac Surg 1998; 27: 315-320.

[30] Bajpai P K. Biodegradable scaffolds in orthopedic, oral and maxillofacial surgery. Rubin L R. Biomaterials in Reconstructive surgery; St. Louis, Mosby, 1983:156

[31] Hutmacher D, Kirsch A, Ackermann KL, Hürzeler MB. Matrix and Carrier Materials for Bone Growth Factors - State of the Art and Future Perspectives in: Stark GB, Horch R, Tancos E(eds). Biological Matrices and Tissue Reconstruction, Springer Verlag, Heidelberg, Germany, 1998; p197-206

[32] Shikinami Y, Okuno M. Bioresorbable devices made of forged composites of hydroxyapatite (HA) particles and poly-L-lactide (PLLA): Part I. Basic characteristics. Biomaterials, 20:859-877, 1998
[33] Vieth WR. Diffusion in and through Polymers: Principles and Applications., Carl Hanser Verlag, München 1991
[34] Tom JW, Debenedetti PG. Particle Formation with Supercritical Fluids – A Review. J Aerosol Sci., 1991; Vol 22, No5, pp 555-584
[35] Michaeli W., Seibt S., Molding of resorbable polymers at low temperatures, ANTEC 1995, pp.3397-3399.
[36] Hutmacher D. unpublished data
[37] Becker W, Dahlin C, Becker BE, Lekholm U, van Steenberghe D, Higuchi K, Kultje C. The use of e-PTFE membranes for bone promotion around titanium implants placed into extraction sockets: A prospective multicenter study. Int J Oral Maxillofac Implants 1994;9:31-40.
[38] Callan DP. Guided tissue regeneration without a stage 2 surgical procedure: Int J Periodont Rest Dent 1993; 13: 173-179
[39] Nevins M, Mellonig JT. The advantages of localized ridge augmentation prior to implant placement: A staged event. Int J Periodont Rest Dent 1994; 97-111
[40] Zitzmann NU, Naef R, Schärer P. Resorbable Membranes in Combination with BioOss for Guided Bone Regeneration. Int J Oral Maxillofac Implants 1997; 12:844-852.
[41] Jovanovic SA, Schenk RK, Orsini M, Kenney EB. Supracrestal bone formation around dental implants: An experimental dog study. Int J Oral Maxillofac Implants 10:23-31 (1995).
[42] Tinti C, Vincenzi G, Whitely N, Nicolis A. Expanded PTFE titanium reinforced membranes for regeneration of mucogingival defects. J Periodontol 65:1088-1094 (1994).
[43] Simion M, Trisi P, Piatelli A. Vertical ridge augmentation using a membrane technique associated with osseointegrated implants. Int J Periodont Restorative Dent 14:497-511 (1994).
[44] Simion M, Trisi P, Maglione M, Piatelli A. A preliminary report on a method for studying the permeability of expanded polytetrafluoroethylene membrane to bacteria in vitro: A scanning electron microscopic and histological study. J Periodontol 1994;65:755-761.
[45] Nowzari H, Slots J. Microbiologic and clinical study of polytetrafluoroethylene membranes for guided bone regeneration around implants. Int J Oral Maxillofac Implants 1995;10:67-73.
[46] Hürzeler MB, Strub JR. Guided bone regeneration around exposed implants: a new bioresorbable device and bioresorbable membrane pins. Practical Periodontics Aesth Dentistry 1995; 7(10):37-47.
[47] Hutmacher DW, Kirsch, A., Ackermann, KL, Huerzeler, MB. A Tissue Engineered Cell Occlusive Device for Hard Tissue Regeneration – A Preliminary Report. Int J Periodontics Restorative Dentistry (in press)

Dietmar W. Hutmacher,[1,2] Swee H. Teoh,[1] Iwan Zein,[1] Kee Woei Ng,[1] Jan-Thorsten Schantz,[1] and Johanna C. Leahy[3]

Design and Fabrication of a 3D Scaffold for Tissue Engineering Bone

---

Reference: Hutmacher, D. W., Teoh S. H., Zein, I., Ng, K. W., Schantz, J. T., and Leahy, J. C. **"Design and Fabrication of a 3D Scaffold for Tissue Engineering Bone,"** *Synthetic Bioabsorbable Polymers for Implants, STP 1396,* C. M. Agrawal, J. E. Parr, and S. T. Lin, Eds., American Society for Testing and Materials, West Conshohocken, PA, 2000.

Abstract: Autogenous cell transplantation is one of the most promising new techniques being developed for bone generation as it eliminates problems of donor site scarcity, immune rejection and pathogen transfer. Osteoblasts obtained from an individual patient can be grown in culture and seeded onto a three-dimensional scaffold that will slowly degrade and resorb as the bone or cartilage structures grow and assimilate in vivo. The three-dimensional (3D) scaffold provides the necessary support for cells to maintain their differentiated state and defines the overall shape of the new bone and cartilage. The necessity of using a scaffold structure as the basic template of engineering tissues has encouraged the study the application of advanced manufacturing technologies in this field. For example, rapid prototyping (RP) technologies such as fused deposition modeling (FDM) can be used to fabricate complex 3D structures based on two-dimensional (2D) cross-sectional data obtained by slicing a computer-aided design (CAD) models. FDM is currently being applied in our laboratory to fabricate bioresorbable 3D scaffolds of various porosities and micro-architecture for tissue engineering bone.

Keywords: Tissue engineering, bioresorbable 3D scaffolds, fused deposition modeling

Introduction

Different processing techniques have been developed to produce scaffolds for tissue engineering bone [*1,2*]. Conventional techniques for scaffold fabrication

---

[1]Laboratory for Biomedical Engineering, National University of Singapore, 10 Kent Ridge Crescent, Singapore 119260

[2] Department of Orthopedic Surgery, National University of Singapore, 10 Kent Ridge Crescent, Singapore 119260

[3] Department for Mechanical and Production Engineering, National University of Singapore, 10 Kent Ridge Crescent, Singapore 119260

include fiber bonding, solvent casting, particulate leaching, membrane lamination and melt molding. Ideally, a scaffold should: (i) be three-dimensional and highly porous with an interconnected pore network for cell growth and flow transport of nutrients and metabolic waste, (ii) be biocompatible and bioresorbable with controllable degradation rate to match tissue replacement, (iii) have suitable surface chemistry for cell attachment and proliferation, and (iv) have mechanical properties to match those of the tissues at the site of implantation.[*2*] The characteristics of scaffolds made from traditional polymer-processing techniques can be similarly produced using rapid prototyping technologies with highly controlled and reproducible porosity and 3D micro-architecture.[*3,4*] In addition, this technology offers the ease and flexibility of varying the scaffold characteristics to meet specific structural and functional requirements of the tissue of interest.

Rapid prototyping (RP) requires the use of specialized software such as Quickslice (QS) (Stratasys Inc. (Eden Prairie, MN) to generate geometrical information from which an RP machine can create a 3D physical model. The geometrical data can be generated from parameters which are inputted directly into the QS program (.SLC format), or by using the software to segment a 3D CAD model into thin slices or layers (.SDL format). Both these methods result in 2D slice data which can be automatically converted into a format (.SML); this data is then used to generate instructions on the form of build paths to enable the RP machine to manufacture a 3D object layer by layer.

Multidisciplinary research teams have previously used various RP technologies to produce artificial limbs, prosthetic implants, and surgical-planning models of internal body structures [*5*]. For the purpose of producing scaffolds for tissue engineered implants, the layered manufacturing process allows different strata within the geometrical structure to have different scaffold characteristics.Fused deposition modeling (FDM) is currently being used by our group to fabricate scaffolds of various porosities and micro-architecture. The process involves the extrusion of a polymer filament through a heated nozzle and deposition of the molten material as thin layers on a platform, as shown schematically in Figure 1. The research project described in this paper focused on the application of poly(caprolactone) (PCL) to fabricate bone scaffold structures using fused deposition modeling.

Poly(caprolactone) is a semicrystalline, biodegradable polymer belonging to the aliphatic polyesters family. The ester group is responsible for the chemical degradability of the polymer through hydrolysis [3]. PCL is used in Capronor, a one-year implantable subdermal contraceptive device [*6*] and in bioresorbable Monocryl monofilament sutures [*7*]. Extensive in-vitro and in-vivo biocompatibilty and efficacy studies have been performed, resulting in FDA approval of these products; PCL is currently regarded as a non-toxic and tissue-compatible material [8]. It was selected over other aliphatic polyesters for FDM because of its favorable properties for thermoplastic processing. It has a low T_g of –60°C, T_m of 60°C and a high decomposition temperature of 350°C [9], with a wide range temperatures which allow extrusion. It also has one of the slowest degradation rates of all biodegradable polymers [10], thus it is the best candidate for fabricating scaffolds to be used in engineering tissues that require a scaffold matrix with extended degradation and resorption kinetics.

This study describes how FDM was used to fabricate PCL scaffolds of various porosities and micro-architecture. It also details how these scaffolds were assessed, qualitatively and quantitatively, using scanning electron microscopy (SEM), mechanical testing, gas permeation chromatography and differential scanning calorimetry (DSC). The efficacy of such PCL scaffolds for tissue culturing was also investigated.

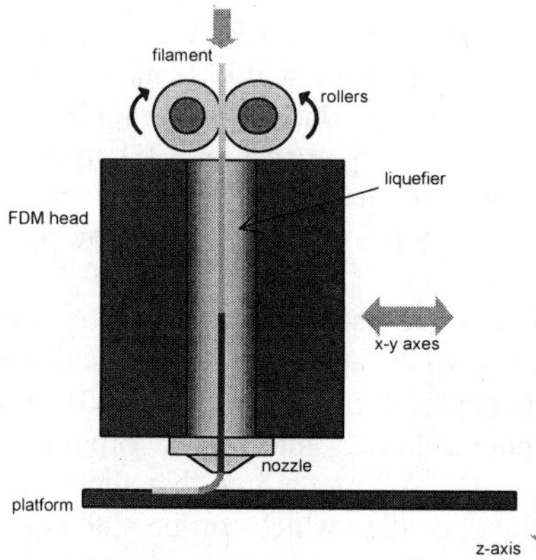

Figure 1 – *Schematic drawing of the computer-controlled FDM process. Thermoplastic polymer filaments are fed into a so called 'liquefier head' via rollers. The head rides in the horizontal x and y-axis. The fixtureless build platform moves in the z-axis. The filament softens and melts inside the liquefier by applying a temperature slightly above the polymers melting temperature. The rollers transport the incoming filament, resulting in a small positive force which drives the extrusion of the melted polymer material. The filament itself acts as a piston extruder in addition to its feed material function.*

Materials and Methods

Materials

Pellets of polycaprolactone (catalog no. 44,074-4) from Aldrich Chemical Company, Inc. (Milwaukee, WI) were used for this study. This semi-crystalline biodegradable polymer has an average M_n of ca. 80,000 (GPC) with a melt index of 1.0g/10min (ASTM D1238-73). It has a melting point of 60°C (DSC). The polymer pellets were kept in a dessicator prior to usage.

Filament Fabrication

Filament fabrication was performed using a fiber-spinning machine (Alex James & Associates Inc., Greensville, SC). Polymer pellets were melted at 190°C in a cylinder by an external heating jacket. After a hold-time of 15 min, the temperature was lowered to 140°C and the polymer melt was extruded through a spinerette with a die exit diameter of 0.064" (1.63mm). Each batch of PCL pellets weighed 30 ± 1g. The piston speed was set at 10mm/min. The extrudate was quenched in chilled water placed 40mm below the die exit. The combination of temperature, piston speed and height-drop to water quenching settings produced a filament diameter of 1.70 ± 0.10mm. The PCL filaments were fabricated to have a consistent diameter to fit the drive wheels of an unmodified FDM system. The filaments were vacuum-dried and kept in a dessicator prior to usage.

Scaffold Fabrication

Scaffold specimens were fabricated using PCL filaments with a FDM 3D Modeler rapid prototyping system from Stratasys Inc. (Eden Prairie, MN). Preliminary investigations were carried out to establish the optimum liquefier temperature, roller speed and FDM head speed settings to ensure that, for a particular nozzle tip size, the extruded PCL adhered sufficiently to the platform and also the preceding layers.[4] It was possible to model and manufacture four scaffold specimens simultaneously, so four rectangular prisms each 32.0 (length) × 25.5 (width) × 13.5mm (height) were created directly in the Stratasys' QuickSlice (QS) software in layers of 0.01" (0.254mm) spacing. The head speed, fill gap, and raster angle for every layer were programmed through the QS software and saved as in .SLC the (Slice) file format; Table 1 shows the effect of these parameters on the geometry of the scaffold structures. Two lay-down patterns, 0/90° and 0/60/120°, were used to give a honeycomb-like pattern of square and triangular pores respectively. Gap spacing was varied depending on the FDM tip size to be used during fabrication; for the T16 tip (0.406mm), gap spacing of 0.020" (0.508mm) and 0.028" (0.711mm) was used, for the T10 tip (0.205mm), gap spacing was set at either 0.010" (0.254mm) or 0.016" (0.406mm). This resulted in a total of eight possible scaffold design configurations, as shown in Table 2.

Table 1 - *Scaffold characteristics resulting from setting of different FDM build parameters.*

FDM Build Parameters	Scaffold Characteristics
Road width of rasters	Wall thickness
Fill gap between rasters	Vertical-channel width
Slice thickness	Horizontal-channel width
Raster angle	3D micro-architecture

Table 2. *This shows the eight different configurations of scaffold design created by varying tip size, angle of lay-down pattern and the size of gap space.*

Tip	T16				T10			
Angle	0/90		0/60/120		0/90		0/60/120	
Gap Space (mm)	0.508	0.711	0.508	0.711	0.254	0.406	0.254	0.406

The 2D slice data were converted into QS's .SML (Stratasys Machine Language) file format which automatically generated the build paths based on the input parameters for each slice layer. The .SML data was sent to the FDM machine to fabricate the scaffold specimens using the T16 and T10 tips. The roller speed was set at 60% online loading via the FDM hardware control. The liquefier temperature was set at 120°C and the envelope temperature remained at 25 ± 2°C (ambient temperature) throughout the fabrication process. Figure 2 shows a flow chart, which provides an overview of the process of scaffold fabrication.

After manufacture, the four specimens of each configuration were cut with a very sharp blade into slightly smaller blocks with dimensions 28.0 (length) × 21.0 (width) × 13.5mm (height). One each of these new blocks was used to measure the porosity of the design and then all four specimens were each divided into twelve small scaffold specimens (6.5 x 6.5 x 13.5mm) for microscopical characterization and compression testing, as described in the following sections.

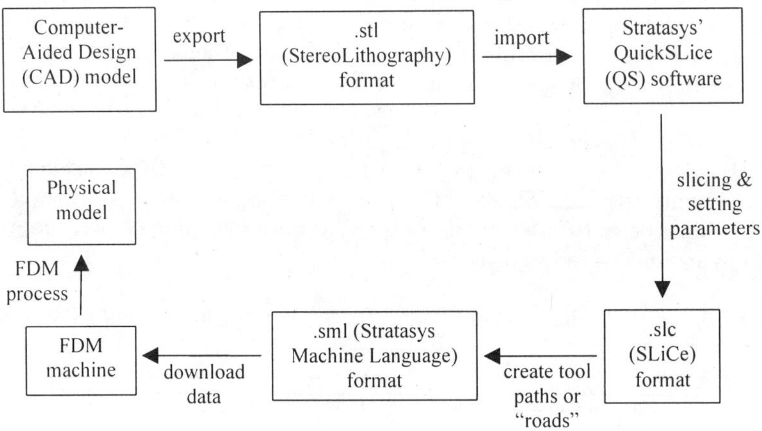

Figure 2 - *Flow chart of data preparation for FDM process*

Porosity Calculation

The ratio of the apparent volume to the true volume of the scaffolds was used to calculate the porosity of each design configuration. An ultrapycnometer (Quantachrome Ultrapycnometer 1000, Quantachrome Corporation, Boynton Beach, FL) was used to measure the true volume of the blocks (28.0 × 21.0 × 13.5mm) at 25°C in pure argon; three measurements were made on each specimen and the mean was used in the porosity calculations. The apparent volume of the blocks was calculated from measurements of their external dimensions, made using digital vernier calipers.

Microscopical Characterization

One each of the scaffold specimens measuring 6.5 × 6.5 × 13.5mm was used to measure the pore size of the scaffold on scanning electron microscopy (SEM) photographs. The methods of preparation of the specimens varied depending on the tip size employed during fabrication on the FDM machine. The T16 specimens were freeze-fractured after dipping in liquid nitrogen for 30min. The T10 specimens could not be freeze-fractured so instead were cut with a sharp blade. All the cut and fracture surfaces were then gold sputtered using a JEOL fine coater JFC-1200 at 10mA for12s. These were studied using a JEOL scanning electron microscope JSM-5800LV operating at 15kV.

Compression Testing

The compressive mechanical properties of the scaffold specimens manufactured with the T16 tip were measured using an Instron 4502 Uni-axial Testing System with 1kN load-cell (Instron Corporation, Canton, MA), following the guidelines set in ASTM F451-99a Standard Specification for Acrylic Bone Cement. This is the latest edition of the same standard used by three other groups [11-13] in their assessment of the mechanical properties of bioresorbable scaffolds for tissue engineering bone.

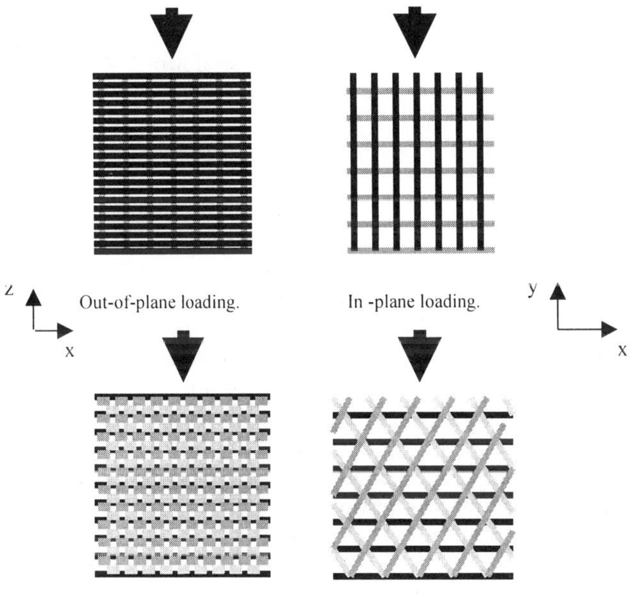

Figure 3 - *Schematic diagram of scaffold structure of a 0/90° (top row) and a 0/60/120° (bottom row) lay-down pattern oriented in different directions such that the loading is out-of-plane or in-plane, denoted by the bold arrows with respect to the x-y-z axes of the FDM build process, where each plane contains one layer of deposited "roads" in a particular direction.*

Due to the nature of the FDM process in its highly directional deposition of materials, it was hypothesized that the scaffolds would exhibit anisotropic behaviour when compressed in different planes. To test this hypothesis, samples of the same porosity and lay-down pattern were compressed in two directions which were normal to each other. These were defined as in-plane compression and out-of-plane compression. In-plane compression takes place when the scaffold is aligned such that the direction of loading is parallel to the plane which contains filaments deposited in uniform direction, i.e. in the x-y plane of the FDM build process. Out-of-plane compression takes place when the scaffold is aligned with the direction of loading normal to the plane which contains filaments deposited in uniform direction, i.e. in the z-direction of the FDM build process. Figure 3 illustrates the in-plane and out-of-plane loading of a FDM scaffold. Ten samples (6.5 x 6.5 x 13.5mm) of each design configuration were tested by loading both in-plane (n = 5) and out-of-plane (n = 5).

The specimens were compressed at a rate of 1mm/min up to a strain-level of approximately 0.7mm/mm; the load-deformation curve was recorded throughout. The Young's modulus (MPa) was calculated, from the stress-strain curve, as the slope of the initial linear portion of the curve, neglecting any toe region due to initial settling of the specimen. Compressive strength at yield was defined as the intersection of the stress-strain curve with the modulus slope at an offset of 1.0% strain.

Gas Permeation Chromatography

The polymer molecular weight distribution was determined by gel permeation chromatography equipped with a differential refractor (Waters, Model 410, Milford, MA) and an absorbance detector refractor (Waters, Model 2690, Milford, MA). The samples were dissolved in tetrahydrofuran (THF) and eluted in a series of configuration through a Styragel columns refractor (Waters, Milford, MA) at a flow rate of $1mlmin^{-1}$. Polystyrene standards (Polysciences, Warrington, PA) were used to obtain a calibration curve.

Differential Scanning Calorimetry

A thermal analysis differential scanning calorimeter (TA Instruments DSC 2910, New Castle, DE) was utilized to analyze the thermal transition of the PCL samples during melting to measure the crystallinity fraction. PCL samples were extracted at stages of filament and scaffold fabrication and were represented by the raw PCL pellet, melt-extruded PCL filament and the extruded "roads" from FDM tip sizes T10 and T16. Samples of 7.0 to 7.7mg were heated at a rate of $5^{o}C$/min from $25^{o}C$ to 70° in aluminum pans under nitrogen. The crystallinity fractions were based upon an enthalpy of fusion value of 139.5J/g for 100% crystalline PCL as reported.[14]

Cell Harvest and Culture

Primary human bone marrow cells were isolated and characterized according to the methods described for bone ex-plant cultures. [15] Monolayer cell culture flasks were filled with 3 to 5 small pieces of bone marrow from the iliac crest of a 5 year old patient and culture media 199 supplemented with 10% fetal bovine serum, 1% peniclin, and 1% streptomycin and 1% amphoterecin. Then the flasks were placed in an self-sterilizable incubator (WTB Binder, Tuttlingen, Germany) at 37 ^{o}C in 5% CO_2, 95% air, and 99% relative humidity.

After the monolayer-culture grew to confluence and exhibited nodule formation, the osteoblasts were harvested using a 0,05% trypsinethylendiamine tetra-acetic acid (EDTA) solution, split, resuspended in culture medium and filled into new culture flasks. The culture media was replaced every third or fourth day. The osteoblastic-phenotype was verified by alkaline phosphatase and osteocalcin staining. [16]

Scaffold Seeding and Culture

In order to investigate the efficacy of PCL scaffolds for tissue culturing, the fabrication techniques previously described were used to manufacture scaffold specimens measuring, 8 x 8 x 5mm. Twelve PCL scaffolds with a 0/60/120° lay-down pattern and two different porosities (48% and 61 %) were assessed. After the fourth passage osteoblast cultures were trypsinized and cell viability was examined via trypan blue (Sigma, StLouis, MO) exclusion. Viable cells were impermeable to trypan blue, whereas non-viable cells were permeable. A 10 ml of trypan blue cell solution is pippeted on a hemocytometer (cells ml $^{-1}$) and viable cells were counted using phase contrast microscopy (10 x objective). The cell concentration was 4 x 10^7 cells ml $^{-1}$. The scaffolds were seeded with 2 x 10^7 cells/scaffold. A 0,5 ml fibrin glue suspension (Immuno, Heidelberg, Germany) was added on each scaffold. The establishment of the osteoblast-like phenotype and intercellular connections were examined daily by phase-contrast light microscopy for two weeks. Adhesion of the cells and their distribution was studied via environmental scanning electron microscopy (ESEM).

Results and Discussion

Porosity Calculation and Microscopical Characterization

Porosity of the scaffolds ranged from 47.6 ± 0.1% to 60.7 ± 0.1% and from 68.6 ± 0.1% to 74.4 ± 0.1% for the T16 and T10 scaffold specimens respectively. The pore size measured based on SEM micrographs fell within the range of 240 - 690μm for the T16 set and 330 - 670μm for the T10 set.

The structure of the scaffolds designed and fabricated using the FDM method were highly similar to the honeycomb of the bee, with its regular array of identical pores, when viewed in the z-direction of the fabrication process. The FDM scaffolds fabricated had two distinctive patterns: one with square pores as a result of a 0/90° lay-down pattern; the other with triangular pores as a result of a 0/60/120° lay-down pattern. Both lay-down patterns can be clearly observed using SEM as seen in Figures 4(a-d).

The main difference lies in the shape of the pores: the bee's honeycomb comprises of hexagonal pores surrounded by solid faces/walls which nest together to fill a plane, but the FDM scaffold structure is built from inter-crossing filaments stacked in horizontal planes and comprises of pores surrounded by solid edges/struts. Even though the pores of the bee's honeycomb are usually hexagonal in section, they can also be triangular, square, or of other polygonal shape in man-made honeycombs [16]; the mechanics of honeycombs lends great understanding to how the FDM scaffolds behave under loading forces

Compression Testing

Figure 5 shows a typical stress-strain curve for a PCL scaffold specimen. This curve demonstrates the typical behaviour of a honeycomb undergoing deformation. It comprises of three distinct regions: a linear-elastic region followed by a plateau of roughly constant stress, leading into a final region of steeply rising stress. Table 3 shows the results obtained from compression testing of the scaffolds.Statistical analysis of the results was used to compare the stiffness and the compressive yield strength of the different configurations of T16 scaffolds, as explained in the following sections. A Student's t-test for independent variables was used to check for differences between results obtained for different designs, after normality, which is a prerequisite for using the t-test, had been established using an Andersen-Darling test. [17] Figure 6 provides a comparative overview of the results.

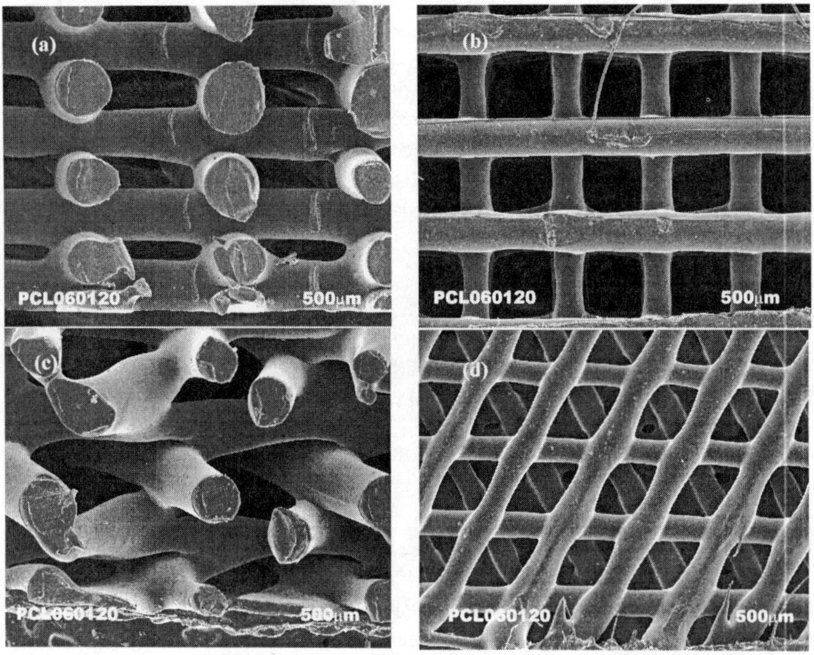

Figure 4a-d - *Freeze-fractured surfaces of two T16 PCL scaffolds with a 0/90° lay-down pattern, porosity 53% (a) side view, (b), top view and with a 0/60/120° lay-down pattern, porosity 61% (c) top view, (d) side view. View of PCL scaffold in the –z direction of the FDM build process of a (a) 0/90° lay-down pattern, and (c) 0/60/120° lay-down pattern, showing a honeycomb pattern with square and triangle pores respectively.*

In-plane compression. When compressed in-plane, the pore edges/struts first bear the loading stress. On first loading they bend, demonstrating linear elasticity as PCL itself is linear-elastic. But when a critical stress level is reached the pores begin to collapse with elastic buckling of the pore edges/struts. Eventually, at high strains, the pores collapse sufficiently to allow adjacent edges/struts to touch and further deformation compresses the scaffold material itself. This manifests itself as the final, steeply rising portion of the stress-strain curve (Figure 5), also defined as *densification*. [16]

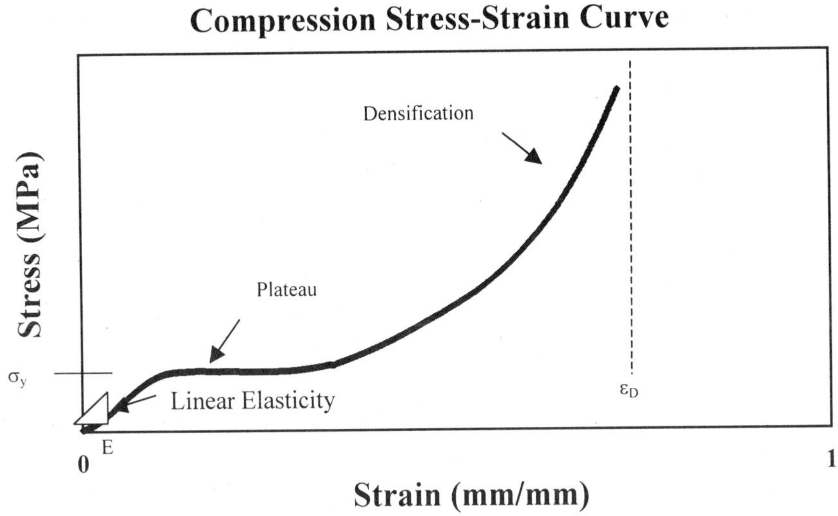

Figure 5 - *A typical compression stress-strain curve of a PCL scaffold fabricated via the FDM method. It is similar to that of a typical honeycomb showing three distinct regions.*

Table 3 *Compressive modulus and compressive yield strength of PCL scaffolds fabricated using a FDM T16 nozzle tip (standard deviation denoted as ± values)*

Lay-down Pattern (°)	Porosity (%)	Compressive stiffness (MPa) (n = 5)		Compressive yield strength (MPa), (n = 5)	
		Out-of-plane	In-plane	Out-of-plane	In-plane
0/90	53	56.6 ± 6.9	77.0 ± 7.6	2.87 ± 0.19	4.05 ± 0.50
0/90	61	44.5 ± 3.3	60.8 ± 8.2	2.51 ± 0.15	3.16 ± 0.52
0/60/120	48	53.8 ± 2.9	53.7 ± 9.5	3.06 ± 0.15	3.89 ± 1.16
0/60/120	61	38.7 ± 3.2	37.6 ± 8.8	2.22 ± 0.09	2.43 ± 0.35

For PCL scaffolds with 53% porosity and a 0/90° lay-down pattern a compressive yield strength and a compressive stiffness of 4.05 ± 0.50 MPa and 77.0 ± 7.6 MPa were found respectively. These values are higher than those of a 61% porous scaffold of the same lay-down pattern. The 0/60/120° lay-down pattern scaffolds also exhibited a similar trend; the 48% porous scaffold having a significantly higher ($p \leq 0.05$) stiffness and yield strength values (53.7 ± 9.5 and 3.89 ± 1.16 MPa) than the 61% porous scaffold

(37.6 ± 8.8 and 2.43 ± 0.35 MPa). The greater stiffness and yield strength of the less porous scaffolds is thought to be because the higher the porosity of a scaffold, the larger the pore volume with fewer pore edges/struts per unit volume to bear the compressive load.

Only two sets of scaffolds with the same porosity (61%) were compared to check the effect of different lay-down pattern on the compressive properties of the scaffold. The scaffolds with a $0/90^{\circ}$ lay-down pattern had a significantly higher compressive stiffness and yield strength than those with a $0/60/120^{\circ}$ lay-down pattern ($p \leq 0.05$). This was most likely due to the alignment of the pore edges/struts with respect to the loading direction. The scaffolds with a $0/90^{\circ}$ lay-down pattern had more pore edges/struts (every alternate layer) aligned parallel to the loading direction than those with a $0/60/120^{\circ}$ lay-down pattern (every three layers) as shown previously in Figure 4b. The struts are more effective in withstanding deformation when they are loaded axially than at an inclination.

Out-of-plane compression - When compressed out-of-plane, it is the intersection points of the pore edges/struts that first bear the loading stress. The initial linear-elastic deformation involves significant shear deformation of the pore edges/struts themselves. In compression, the linear-elastic regime is truncated by elastic buckling and final failure is by crushing of the pore edges/struts of adjacent planes.

Statistical analysis again confirmed that scaffolds of higher porosity had significantly lower stiffness and yield strengths under compression loading than those of lower porosity ($p \leq 0.05$). The 61% porous scaffold had lower compressive stiffness and yield strength than the 53% porous scaffold because it had larger pore volume and consequently less intersection points of the pore edges/struts per unit volume to bear the compressive load. The highest compressive yield strength of 2.87 ± 0.19 MPa was attained for PCL scaffolds with a 53% porosity and a $0/90^{\circ}$ lay-down pattern. The highest compressive stiffness of 56.6 ± 6.9 MPa was attained for PCL scaffolds with a 53% porosity and a $0/90^{\circ}$ lay-down pattern. These values were higher than those of 61% porous scaffold of the same lay-down pattern. The $0/60/120^{\circ}$ lay-down pattern scaffolds also exhibited the same trend, with the 48% porous scaffold having higher compressive stiffness and yield strength than the 61% porous scaffold (Student's t-test, $p \leq 0.05$).

Two sets of scaffolds with 61% porosity were compared to check the effect of varying the lay-down pattern on the compressive properties of the scaffold in out-of-plane testing. The scaffolds with a $0/90^{\circ}$ lay-down pattern had a significantly higher compressive stiffness and yield strength than those with a $0/60/120^{\circ}$ lay-down pattern ($p \leq 0.05$), but to a lesser extent than those for in-plane loading.

Comparison between the in-plane and out-of-plane properties - The scaffolds with a $0/90^{\circ}$ lay-down pattern were found to be significantly stiffer and stronger when loaded in the direction parallel to the plane containing filaments of uniform direction ($p \leq 0.05$). However, the scaffolds with a $0/60/120^{\circ}$ lay-down pattern did not show any statistical difference in the properties when tested in-plane and out-of-plane ($p > 0.05$). It can be concluded that scaffolds with the $0/60/120^{\circ}$ lay-down pattern do not exhibit anisotropic behavior to the same extent as their counterparts with $0/90^{\circ}$ lay-down pattern.

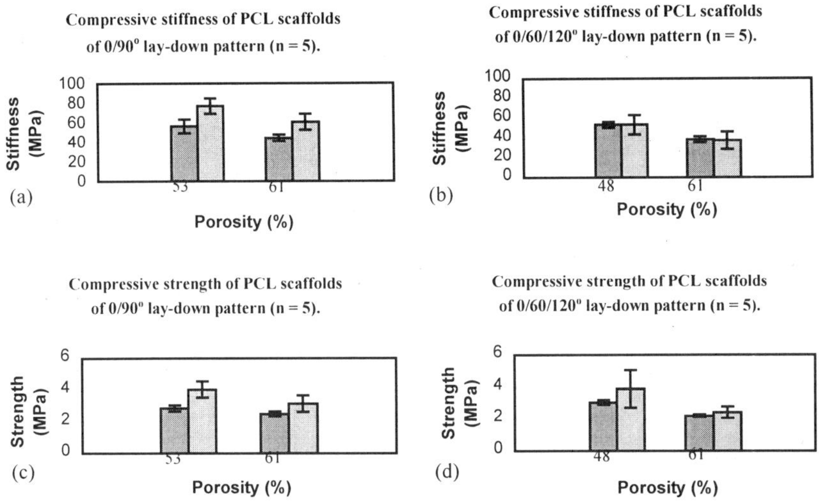

Figure 6 - *Compressive stiffness of (a) 0/90° lay-down pattern and (b) 0/60/120° lay-down pattern PCL scaffolds. Compressive yield strength at 1.0% strain of (c) 0/90° lay-down pattern and (d) 0/60/120° lay-down pattern PCL scaffolds. Error bars denote ± S.D. for n =5. The porosity was calculated based on true volume measurement using an ultrapycnometer.*

Differential Scanning Calorimetry

The crystallinity fraction of PCL was not observed to rise significantly when the polymer was processed into filaments via the melt-extrusion process and subsequently through the FDM process. The values ranged between 56% to 58%. The shear forces on the polymer melt during the filament extrusion as well as FDM processes did not cause the percentage of crystallites to change significantly.

Table 4 *DSC results for different PCL specimens.*

PCL sample (n =2)	Crystallinity fraction (%)		
	sample 1	sample 2	average
Raw pellet	54.1	57.7	55.9
Raw filament	59.7	56.2	58.0
T10 scaffold	57.5	57.0	57.3
T16 scaffold	58.8	57.7	58.3

Gas Permeation Chromatography

The degradation of PCL by the melt processing methods, filament extrusion and fused deposition modeling was characterized by measuring the molecular weight. The results of the gas permeation chromatography (GPC) are shown in Table 3. The processing temperatures did not result in a significant change of the molecular weight.

Table 5 *Molecular weight distribution of the different specimens.*

PCL sample	M_n	M_w	Polydispersity M_w / M_n
Raw pellet	78,542	139,923	1.781500
Raw filament	82,245	141,359	1.718753
Scaffold S5-8, T10	87,343	146,739	1.680030
Scaffold S5-3, T16	91,990	150,515	1.636216
Scaffold S5-6, T16	84,038	143,765	1.710723

Scaffold Seeding and Culture

Osteoblast-like cells showed a three-dimensional phenotype and established their filipodias and intercellular connections within the fibrin glue matrix and on the PCL scaffolds (Figure 7a-c, 8). The fibrin coating supported an initial cell proliferation and subsequent differentiation to establish a stable matrix structure within a highly porous PCL scaffold. The cell mortality was less than 5% as shown by trypan blue staining and maintained a stable cell metabolism. The cells were able to migrate and differentiate on the PCL surface as well as in the fibrin environment and secreted extracellullar matrix which was subsequently mineralized.[*16*]

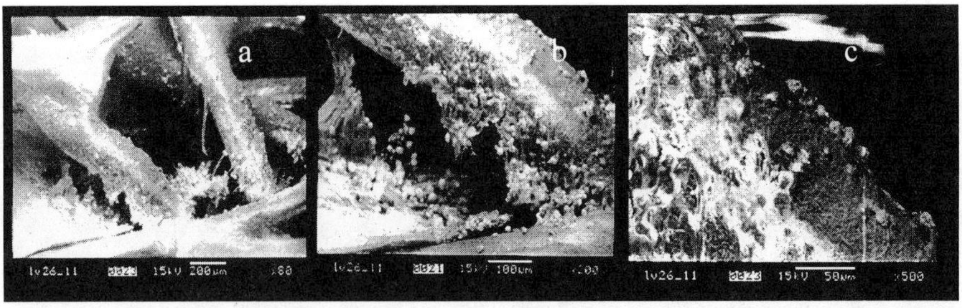

Figure 7 – *Environmental scanning electron microscopy pictures 14 days after seeding with osteoblast-like cells and coating with fibrin glue of a PCL scaffolds (8x8x5mm) with a 0/60/120° lay-down pattern a porosity of 61 %*

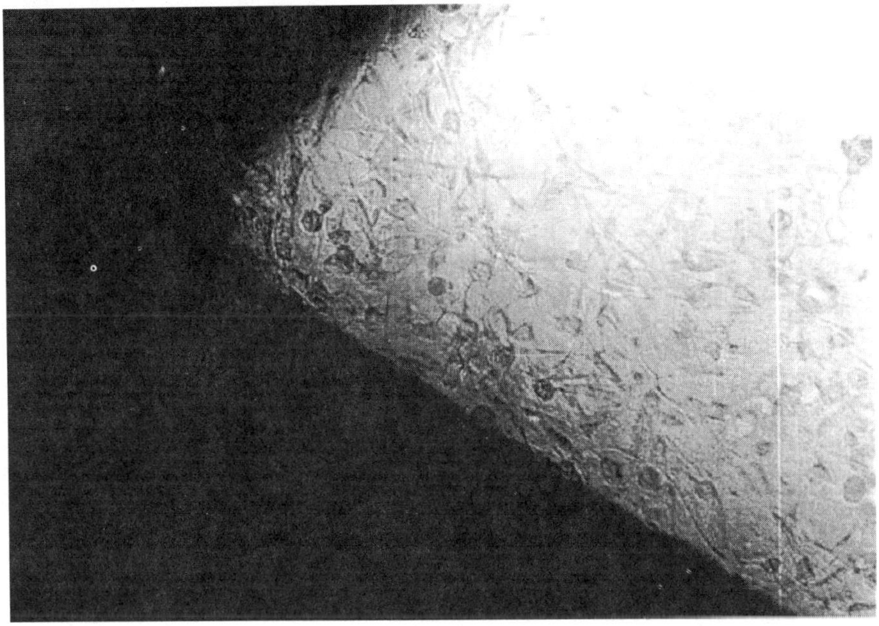

Figure 8 – *Phase-contrast light microscopy 7 days after seeding with osteoblast-like cells and coating with fibrin glue of a PCL scaffolds (8x8x5mm) with a 0/60/120° lay-down pattern a porosity of 61 %*

Conclusion

A highly reproducible and computer-controlled method to design and fabricate porous, bioresorbable 3D scaffolds using fused deposition modeling was developed. The pore volume and structure, and the porosity of the scaffolds, were mainly defined by the setting of the computer-controlled FDM machine parameters. The honeycomb design resulted in similar mechanical properties to cancellous bone [18] and has therefore the potential to be applied in load-bearing applications. However, the mechanical properties of the scaffold need to be further evaluated under physiological testing conditions. Preliminary cell culture studies, using human osteoblasts, showed that a by FDM fabricated PCL matrix has the potential to be used as scaffold material for tissue engineering bone.

References

[1] Widmer M.S., Mikos A.G., Fabrication of Biodegradable Polymer Scaffolds for Tissue Engineering. In Patrick Jr. C.W., Mikos A.G., and McIntire L.V. (eds). Frontiers in Tissue Engineering, Elsevier Science Inc., New York, USA, 1998, pp.107-120.

[2] Hutmacher D., Kirsch A., Ackermann K.L., Huerzeler M.B., Matrix and Carrier Materials for Bone Growth Factors - State of the Art and Future Perspectives. In: Stark G.B., Horch R., Tancos E.(eds).Biological Matrices and Tissue Reconstruction, Springer Verlag, Heidelberg, Germany, 1998, pp.197-206 .

[3] Cima L.G., Vacanti J.P., Vacanti C., Ingber D., Mooney D. and Langer R., Tissue Engineering by Cell Transplantation Using Degradable Polymer Substrates, Journal of Biomechanical Engineering, Vol.113, 1991, pp.143-151.

[4] Zein I, Hutmacher DW, Teoh SH. Bioresorbable Polymer Scaffolds for Tissue Engineering Using an Advanced Manufacturing Technology. 8th Asian Pacific Confederation of Chemical Engineering, Seoul, Korea, 16-19 August 1999, pp 1137-1140.

[5] Ashley S. (ed.), "Rapid prototyping for artificial body parts", Mechanical Engineering, May 1993 pp.50-53.

[6] Darney P.D., Monroe S.E., Klaisle C.M. and Alvarado A., "Clinical evaluation of the Capronor contraceptive implant: preliminary report", American Journal of Obstetrics & Gynecology, 160, 1989, pp.1292-1295.

[7] Bezwada R.S., Jamiolkowski D.D., Lee I., Vishvaroop A., Persivale J., Treka-Benthin S., Erneta M., Suryadevara J., Yang A., and Liu S., "Monocryl suture, a new ultra-pliable absorbable monofilament suture", Biomaterials, 16, 1995, pp.1141-1148,.

[8] Pitt C.G., Schindler A., "Biodegradation of Polymers", Bruck S.D. (ed.), Controlled Drug Delivery, CRC Press, Boca Raton, FL, pp.55-80, 1983.

[9] Suggs L.J., Mikos A.G., "Synthetic biodegradable polymers for medical applications", Mark J.E. (ed.), Physical Properties of Polymers Handbook, 1996 pp.615-624.

[10] Perrin D.E., English J.P., "Polycaprolactone", Domb A.J., Kost J., Wiseman D.M. (eds.), Handbook of Biodegradable Polymers, 1998, pp.63-77.

[11] Peter S.J., Nolley J.A., Widmer M.S., Merwin J.E., Yaszemski M.J., Yasko A.W., Engel P.S., Mikos A.G., In vitro degradation of a poly(propylene fumarate)/β-tricalcium phosphate composite orthopaedic scaffold, Tissue Engineering, vol.3, no.2, 1997, pp.207-215.

[12] Thomson R.C., Yaszemski M.J., Powers J.M., Mikos A.G., Hydroxyapatite fiber reinforced poly(α-hydroxy ester) foams for bone regeneration, Biomaterials, Vol.19, 1998, pp.1935-1943.

[13] Yoon S.N., Jun J.Y., Tae G.P., A novel fabrication method of macroporous biodegradable polymer scaffolds using gas foaming salt as a porogen additive, Journal of Biomedical Materials Research (Applied Biomat.), 53, 2000, pp.1 – 7.

[14] Crescenze V., Manzini G., Calzolari G., and Borri C., Thermodynamics of fusion of poly-β-propiolactone and poly-ε-caprolactone, comparative analysis of the melting

